The Part-Time Diet Approach

For Full-Time Weight Loss

"A Calorically Controlled Love Story"

John Hogan

ISBN: 978-1-4357-0608-8
Published By Lulu.com
www.lulu.com

Printed in the United States of America

DISCLAIMER

This book is a source of information to help you attain and maintain a healthy weight. It is not intended to treat or cure any disease, and is not intended to be a substitute for the advice and council of your personal health care professional. Any application of the material set forth in the following pages is at the readers' discretion and the reader's sole responsibility. Anyone, especially anyone under the age of eighteen years, embarking on any weight-loss, exercise or fitness program should first seek the advice of a qualified health professional.

About The Author

John Hogan, is a Licensed Physical Therapist who graduated from Temple University in 1982 with a bachelor's degree in Physical Therapy. He also holds a bachelor's degree in Computer Science, which he acquired in 2000, from Chestnut Hill College, located in northwestern Philadelphia. Since graduating from Temple, he has worked in hospitals and clinics in the Philadelphia area and has specialized in outpatient orthopedics.

During this time, it became obvious to John that excess weight caused or aggravated many of the conditions with which his patients suffered, and also that the typical approaches to weight loss made the people who practiced them hot-house orchids. In other words, they could follow the diet as long as they stayed in very controlled settings. However, when they left their self-imposed greenhouse and ventured out into the real world, with all its temptations, their discipline would soon evaporate. From this point, it was just a short trip back into the chaotic world of guilt versus hunger: a world in which hunger wins ninety-nine percent of the time.

For approximately the last twenty years, John has been -informally- verbally explaining and coaching people in an approach designed to break this cycle, an approach that is more robust and practical, and one that actually works in the real world by mitigating the drudgery of daily dieting. The writing of this book was driven by the desire to give the reader this same alternative to the many unrealistic weight-loss systems in the market, and also to save John's breath.

Presently, John is Clinical Director of Rehabilitation at a small private practice in the Philadelphia area, and uses the system in this book to manage his own weight. Comments can be directed to johnh@parttimediet.com.

Contents

About The Author

Preface: The Magic Number Of Calories That Will Put You Into
           Nutritional Nirvana And Why The Inventor Of <u>Daily Dieting</u>
           Should Be Jailed And Forced To <u>Diet Daily</u>

Introduction: The Year Of The Shrinking Pants And The Evolution Of This
           Approach   5

   1. Meet Gloria And See Why Traditional Diets
       Fail: Calories In Versus Calories Out? It's
       Not Quite That Simple.   8

   2. Getting Started: Let's Revisit Gloria And
       Then Forget Everything You Think You Know
       About Dieting   20

   3. Learning To Count Calories Puts Gloria And
       You In Control: Think Checking Account   39

   4. A Basic Guide To Exercise: To Phil's Relief,
       Grunting And Groaning Is Strictly Optional   93

   5. Putting It All Together: Small Steps Can Take
       You Far   127

   6. Maintaining The New You: Gloria, Phil And
       You Already Know How   145

   Appendix A: BMR VALUES   161

   References   204

   Index   205

Preface

The Magic Number Of Calories That Will Put You Into Nutritional Nirvana, And Why The Inventor Of <u>Daily Dieting</u> Should Be Jailed And Forced To <u>Diet Daily</u>

Diet as little as one day per week and lose weight! How is this possible? The answer is simple. It's possible because, for each of us, there is a "magical" number of calories that our body needs to maintain its weight. If you were to eat this number of calories six days per week and, just for discussion's sake, let's say half that number on the seventh day, you would lose weight. Depending on your size, this could be a half-pound per week or more.

Want faster weight loss? Just diet two days per week. Even faster, diet three days per week. Following this sequence to its logical conclusion, we should diet every day for fastest weight-loss, right?

Wrong! Unlike what other weight-loss systems would have you believe, there's more to this puzzle than simple addition and subtraction. The truth is: if you eat less than you need, i.e. diet every day, after some period of time, you will reach the undoing of most diets: the dreaded plateau. You know, you're dieting for a while and weight is falling off like clockwork, and then suddenly, the scale refuses to move, despite your following your program to the letter. Sound familiar? Once this response sets in, it can stop any weight-loss effort cold.

The reason for this conundrum lies in the body's ability to lower its calorie needs in response to lower calorie intake. In other words, in the face of daily calorie restriction, the body adapts and learns to function on less food. The Part-Time Diet Approach mitigates this response by varying the calorie intake on a weekly basis, in effect resetting the body's perception of its calorie needs.

By using this calorie varying technique, a dieter can produce consistent, easy weight-loss and circumvent the dreaded plateau. The dynamic component inherent in the Part-Time Diet Approach also alleviates the daily drudgery and psychological beating that daily dieting causes. A nice side effect of this technique is that from day one, you will also be training yourself to maintain your goal weight when you reach it.

So, if you're interested in learning a step-by-step, nuts and bolts system to lose and manage weight for the rest of your life that requires you to diet on only one to four days per week -The Part-Time Diet Approach actually prohibits daily dieting, and weight-maintenance requires no dieting- requires no special foods, inhuman willpower, motivation, or inspiration then it is my humble opinion that you should read on.

Introduction

The Year Of The Shrinking Pants And *The Evolution Of This Approach*

It was late 1977. "Saturday Night Fever" was number one at the box office, and disco music was at its zenith as a cultural phenomenon. I was 20 years old then, and it seemed I could empty the contents of any fast-food restaurant into my stomach as frequently as I wished, and never gain a pound. Well, maybe not literally, but it sure seemed that way. Then, a scant year later, my seemingly bulletproof metabolism began to betray me, and before the 1980s dawned, my weight ballooned by 35 pounds, and my pants shrank to what my mother called "skin-on-baloney" proportions. Now don't get me wrong, I did not assume victim status and passively go along for the ride. I fought back with all the sundry methods available, including: low-carbohydrate, (yes low-carb was around even then) low-fat, and cutting calories to an untenable minimum. All these methods worked to stem the expansion of my fat cells for a short time, but just as reliably, they all failed over the long-term.

Motivated as much by panic as anything else, I adopted a simple 1500-calories-per-day diet. Following this regimen, I lost three pounds per week and managed to attain my old high school weight. During this time, I exercised religiously and this, no doubt, contributed to my success. Despite all the exercise though, when the scale finally agreed with my internal self-image, the mirror did not. Yes, I looked thinner, but I did not have the lean, muscular look I remembered. It was obvious that I had lost muscle tissue during this process.

No problem. When I was a teenybopper, I had trained to gain muscle. All I had to do was eat a little more and continue to weight-train, so I increased the calories relative to what I was eating during my diet, and pushed the heaviest weights I could handle. After about three months, I found that I did indeed gain some muscle, but at a cost of some regain of body fat. OK, just re-lose the body fat and everything would be copasetic. Uh, not quite that simple because losing weight caused me to, again, lose muscle tissue. Dogged devotion to this approach, despite many efforts to fine-tune it, resulted in my getting weaker and fatter.

Fortunately, during this time, I had documented calories eaten and weight lost on years worth of calendars. One evening, I happened to be looking at these numbers, and I realized that based on these data, I could eat much more than I thought I could without gaining weight. A little math told me that at my current activity level, I should be able to maintain my weight by eating roughly 3000 calories per day. I decided to test this theory, and after three months, it proved to be true. I could indeed eat that many calories per day without gaining a pound. At this point, I had solved half the puzzle, but didn't realize it. By following this rather luxurious regimen, I was able to maintain my weight with little effort. Then it occurred to me that as long as I never exceeded my caloric limit, I could now lose weight by eating some number of calories less than 3000 on just a few days per week. The first iteration of this program simply consisted of cutting my normal food intake in half on just three days per week. So, if I would normally eat two bowls of cereal in the morning, I would just eat one; a tuna sandwich for lunch became a half-sandwich and, well, you get the idea.

When I realized the significance of what I had discovered, I was ecstatic. Essentially, I could adjust my weight without the daily deprivation of the traditional diet. To say I felt empowered is as much an understatement as saying Clark Kent felt "good" when he discovered he could fly. I had hated not being my old self, and finding that I could maintain the old me with only a modicum of self-discipline was like finding the Holy Grail. This technique finally allowed me to lose weight and keep the muscle, and matured into the system espoused in this book.

That was 1985, and since then, I have been informally using the same basic system, albeit a bit more evolved than it was then, to help people attain and, more importantly, maintain weight loss. Over these last twenty-plus years, I, and some of my co-workers, have probably repeated these principles a couple thousand times, so I thought writing it down might make sense. The result of this labor is a book that contains all the tools necessary for readers to accomplish their own weight loss goals.

Just so we're clear, this system does not prohibit or recommend any special foods, requires no tapes, seminars, counseling by "nutrition experts", religious fervor, biochemistry degrees, weekly fees, meal packages or inhuman self-discipline. That means, up to your caloric limit, you can have popcorn at the movies, hot dogs with the bun while watching a baseball game or an opera — what goes better together than hot dogs and the opera — the occasional adult beverage, and the list goes on and on.

To make the system, hopefully, more understandable, I have also created two semi-fictitious characters who will help illustrate exactly how the system might get done in the real world, what to expect during the different stages, and how to use this approach to overcome the obstacles common to any weight-loss endeavor. Their stories, including their occasional missteps, will be intertwined with the explanation of the system, and will hopefully make this the last weight-loss book you will ever need. Enjoy!

1	**Meet Gloria And See Why Traditional Diets Fail**

Calories In Versus Calories Out? It's Not Quite That Simple

With over twenty-five years in the practice of Physical Therapy, you might say that I've seen my share of spinal dysfunction. In the majority of cases, body weight has played a role in the evolution of this problem. Since I and some of my colleagues –the "we" I occasionally refer to throughout this book- have always believed in treating the whole person, we have offered diet and exercise as a way to effect long-term relief from this, as well as other maladies. During this time, it has become obvious that the typical approaches to weight loss are largely ineffective over the long-term. Ineffective, because they contain a fundamental flaw, which I will illustrate in this book. When you know what this flaw is, you will know why approaches like 'just eat 500 calories less than you need each day and you'll lose a pound a week', or 'cut out such and such food', or 'just don't eat four hours before bedtime', are short fixes at best.

That being said, just about all diets work when you first start them. This is why there are so many weight-loss programs on the market, and also why the first days and weeks for most dieters are full of euphoria and a feeling of confidence, no matter which diet they try. These feelings are soon dashed as whatever program they are following begins to lose its effectiveness. At this point, some people just give up, while some redouble their efforts, examine what they are doing, and tighten down on their caloric limit. This usually seems to work, but after a short time, another barrier is encountered, and weight loss stops, or worse, begins to reverse despite one's best efforts. The final leg of this journey ends with the dieter concluding that they cannot lose weight, resuming their old eating habits and regaining all the weight they have lost, plus more.

Ironically, it is the initial success of these types of diet plans that causes people to, after some time, try the same failed diet approach again and again. The thought process is that it is not the plan that failed, but it is they who have failed in their execution of the plan. Since, as much as, one third of the weight lost with these approaches is muscle tissue, and all the weight regained is fat, each time down this path causes you to increase the percentage of your body weight that is composed of fat. This scenario plays out over and over, as thousands of people start diets every day: diets that, after a year's time, are statistically doomed to failure.

Right about now, you are probably starting to wonder why this happens. After all, if you eat less than your body requires every day, shouldn't you lose weight consistently? Virtually anyone who has tried this type of dieting knows that the answer to this question is no, and this fact underlies one of the basic mistakes most diet plans make. That is: they approach dieting as though the body is a static unchanging system. In reality, the body is a mechanism that was designed by nature to respond to, and change with its environment. This change, however, is not instantaneous, and it is during this time when the body is off its feet, so to speak, that we experience the greatest weight loss. This physiological lag time explains the initial rapid weight loss of most diets, because as the body is trying to learn to adapt to the new diet and exercise regimen, it is inefficient. When it is in this phase of adaptation, it uses more calories, and you lose body fat. The Part-Time Diet Approach takes advantage of this fact to keep the body off balance, inefficient and burning calories. It is sort of like starting a new diet every week.

Based on this logic, it is my contention that to achieve consistent body fat loss, we must constantly change our routine and challenge or trick the body into adapting to our eating and exercise habits. It must also be done in a way that requires a minimum of willpower and provides variety in food choices.

Remember, life does not start at the end of some diet; it starts right now, so any realistic weight loss approach must allow you to live a realistic lifestyle. Not only does this approach give you a nuts and bolts system to do this, but it also plans for the resumption of normal eating from day one, so you will be able to maintain your new weight easily, and without sacrificing any of your favorite foods.

One more thought before we begin. Sometimes, we think of losing weight as merely a cosmetic issue, or a pain management issue, but there are many people who have been told by their doctors to lose weight or suffer the consequences of some disease(s) like diabetes, arthritis, stroke, or heart disease. Unfortunately, they are rarely given a reasonable way to accomplish this. Often, the doctor has little or no idea themselves, and offers no advice, or worse, gives the typical advice which revolves around some arbitrary daily calorie limit; one woman who weighed over 250 pounds and was put on a starvation diet of 1200 calories per day comes to mind. Many patients have told us of the stark depression they felt as they left their doctor's office with two options: chronic hunger, or catastrophic illness. It is for these people, especially, that this book was written, in the hope of giving them at least one more option.

Before we delve into the nitty-gritty, as promised, let's meet Gloria. She's the first of two composite characters whose journey we will be following through this tome. As you will see, today's not one of her better days.

Low clouds smeared the sky with a dirty gray patina while they unloaded a cold, steady drizzle. Gloria stood on the hilltop where her beloved husband lay interred for the last two years, in fact, two years to the day. It was November 13th and this day, second only to the day of Hugh's funeral, was the grayest day she could remember. The sky was gray, the trees were gray, even the grass surrendered its normal green and brown hue to this weather-beaten, old black-and-white-photograph world. Enduring the small stings of rain hitting her face, she gazed at her husband's headstone. Even now, she couldn't resist shaking her head as she read the dates on it. A tear rolled down her right cheek as she thought, *'Hugh, why did you have to leave so soon?'*

Of course, Hugh knew of his family's propensity for heart disease, and he had certainly been lectured about his weight by more than one cardiologist. None of this, though, had motivated him to change his lifestyle. Even his first heart attack at the age of 32 was not enough to overcome his capacity for denial. He was always too busy to start an exercise program, or too preoccupied to be cognizant of his caloric intake. The nightmare finally materialized just after he turned 40 years old. The bad genes he had inherited and the bad lifestyle choices he had made exacted their toll and took him from his family, and ultimately led to his beloved Gloria standing in a deserted graveyard on this raw autumn afternoon.

Gloria, however, had not allowed her husband's death to stop her from consulting him when she needed to make big decisions. In fact, today's visit, besides honoring the anniversary of his death, was also to get his opinion of her latest endeavors. She knew it was probably just her being silly, but she felt that she could hear his advice best when she was here at his gravesite.

After self-consciously scanning the deserted graveyard, she began to speak aloud to Hugh's gravestone and the wilderness beyond. She started with a long-overdue apology to Hugh for not being harder on him about his excessive weight. She explained that since she too had been battling an on-again, off-again weight problem all her adult life, she felt it would have been hypocritical for her to have nagged him any more than she did.

Hugh's death had actually made a part of her feel that perhaps it was really futile for anyone to battle a weight problem. After all, hadn't every program she ever tried eventually led her back to her starting weight, plus a little bit more? Add to this, the chronic knee problem she had had since her early twenties had gotten to the point where she couldn't walk any real distance, and permanent weight reduction really did seem futile.

This introspection segued into broaching one of the major decisions she had recently made, namely to have the knee surgery her doctor had been recommending for the last few years. In fact, she told Hugh, it was scheduled within the next three days. She further explained her hope that the surgery would enable her to resume her walking program, and somehow finally solve her weight problem, and more importantly, provide a good example for their children. Although neither child was overweight now, she knew that was no guarantee that they hadn't inherited Hugh's tendency to be overweight, and his predisposition to heart disease. At this point, there was really no way to know since Hugh had not been overweight as a child either. Gloria just knew that losing one or both of her children to premature heart disease was a recurring nightmare of hers, and she was determined to do all she could to avoid that catastrophe.

She then told Hugh she had decided to take a few night courses in computer programming and database management. She further explained that she thought these courses could help her get a badly-needed pay raise, and, since the courses were offered at night, they would not interfere with her job.

When she was done with her side of the dialogue, she sat down on the damp ground and leaned back against the cold, indifferent tombstone. After a few seconds, she closed her eyes and just listened. For a while, the silence was broken only by her own heartbeat and the cold wind soughing through the trees. Putting her hands in her coat pockets and hugging herself against the raw day, she smiled as she thought what a sight she must have made leaning against her husband's tombstone. She couldn't help it, this is where she felt most secure.

After a few minutes, she opened her eyes. The wind had died down, but still provided a background moan over which she thought she heard, no felt, for just a fleeting moment, her husband's soft whisper. She stood and looked all around. She was alone. Probably just the wind tussling the treetops, she thought, but then suddenly, a ray of late afternoon sunlight cleaved the low cloud cover and colorized the preternaturally gray world. Gloria smiled as she felt the warmth of the sun and, she liked to think, of her husband's smile. She would take this ephemeral glimpse of sunlight as her answer. Basking in this perfect peace, she laughed and said, "Hugh, you're so melodramatic."

After a few moments, the wind and drizzle whipped up again as if to chase her downhill to her car. As she drove away, though, the sense of peace she felt before continued to envelop her. Her career and surgical decisions just felt right now, and she felt an almost euphoric optimism about them. That strange optimism also extended to her future battle of the bulge, but it was also accompanied by a pang of concern. Her past experience, with the all-too-temporary results that even her best efforts at losing weight had provided, raised the question: what would be different this time around?

Poor Gloria, fortunately, for her, she's fictitious. Anyway, before we see where Gloria's decisions will take her, let's examine what happens when a person embarks on the typical diet, and why Gloria's efforts have met with only limited and temporary success.

As mentioned before, the first few weeks of practically any diet usually result in weight loss often exceeding the dieter's expectations. Then, at some point, weight loss ceases, and the dieter is said to have hit a plateau. At this point, the dieter goes one of two ways. They either give up and resume their former "sinful" ways, which more often than not causes them to regain all of the weight lost and then some, or they decide to even further limit their intake of food. If the dieter chooses the latter path, they will often resume weight loss, but not at the same rapid pace as when the diet was first started.

Depending on the person's intransigence, some number of these, "eat less, plateau, eat less, plateau" cycles will be endured until they conclude that they are a failure, or they are not good enough to be thin, or (insert your own reason here). Like the dieter who gave up after the first plateau, when they finally resume their former eating habits, weight regain is inevitable.

If this has happened to you, don't feel bad. It has been posited that losing weight, or more precisely, chronically depriving oneself of enough food to create hunger is even harder than quitting smoking. After all, you cannot just stop eating altogether, so you must learn to control one of your most primal urges, an urge that is rooted in your instinct for survival.

Even if you have the iron will power it takes to overcome this physical urge, you may find that chronic and severe caloric restriction can cause other, more emotional, issues with which many chronic dieters are familiar. Anyone who has been down this road knows I am referring to the feelings of deprivation and isolation that are common when you are the only one at the party who cannot indulge a little because you are committed to some program. Once these negative feelings set in, for most of us, it is only a matter of time until the "extreme" resumption of our former ways.

The take-away from this little section is that, for most dieters, the reasons traditional, everyday diets don't work fall into two main categories. The first is a matter of physiology, and the body's ability to adapt to its environment, while the second deals more with psychological reasons with which most people who have tried dieting are intimately familiar. In the remainder of this chapter, I will try to shed some light on how these problems hinder your weight loss efforts, and how you can circumvent them.

The One-Two Punch Of Daily Caloric Deprivation

Before we get started, we need to make sure we are on the same page with regard to what we mean by dieting. For the purposes of this book, we will define dieting as eating fewer calories over a given time period than it takes to maintain your body weight. So, if your body requires 2000 calories per day to maintain your weight and you eat 1500 on a certain day, then you are dieting on that day. If you eat 2000 calories or more on a given day then, on that day, you are not dieting. These numbers can also be viewed within a weekly time frame, so you could say that you would be dieting if you eat less than 14000 (2000 X 7) calories per week. Overeating would, of course, be defined as eating more than 2000 calories in a day or more than 14000 calories in a week. These are simple but important concepts, and they will be used throughout this plan.

Now we all know that chronic overeating leads to weight gain. This is as true a statement as exists in the English language. Since this is so true, it would seem logical to conclude that if you eat less than your body uses, you will lose weight, and, indeed, when you first start a diet, it does work this way. For most of us, though, this initial effectiveness wears off long before we reach our goal weight. In order to understand why this happens, we must first look at things from our body's point of view.

"We are not that long from the cave."

The human body is a dynamic mechanism designed to cope with an ever-changing environment. Numbers often quoted like heart rate, blood pressure, cholesterol, and a plethora of others are constantly changing in response to a host of internal and external environmental conditions. People often quote their blood pressure as if it's cast in stone, never realizing that the very act of speaking raises it. For our purposes, one of the most important of these numbers is the basal metabolic rate (BMR). A good practical definition of this is:

It is the amount of energy you burn when sitting in your favorite chair, not too warm and not too cold, on an empty stomach, while watching a boring television show. Sorry, no munchies allowed, digesting food requires more calories.

Simply put, it is the number of calories your body burns while you are not digesting food, comfortable and at rest, but not sleeping.

The BMR changes in response to many factors, but the main ones are: the number of calories you ingest, the amount of lean body muscle you possess, your age -older people take heart, studies are starting to show that age-related BMR reduction is probably more related to loss of skeletal muscle tissue than to age alone- and your activity level. Simple observation has shown us that if a person chronically eats less than their body needs to maintain weight, at some point, the weight loss just stops. Studies are now starting to show that the loss of so-called fat free body mass (muscle) concomitant with long-term dieting actually slows the BMR to meet the new intake of calories. So, it seems safe to surmise that the first punch of daily dieting hits you square in the metabolism by slowing it down to meet the decreased intake of calories.

This ability to slow the BMR during starvation conditions probably served our ancestors well. Being able to survive on less food undoubtedly contributed to early man becoming present day man. It has been theorized that people today who store body fat easily are probably descended from people who found themselves under starvation conditions frequently. This ability to operate on less food was great for someone lost in the primeval wilderness, but terrible for those of us in the calorically dense, modern culinary forest.

For present day dieters, the body's ability to slow the BMR during lean times creates the aforementioned plateau. Because plateaus can be very stubborn, they are the undoing of many well-intentioned dieters. After one hits a plateau, it may seem, intuitively, that lowering calories further is the answer. Unfortunately, this just brings you to a lower plateau that requires even more self-discipline to maintain or breach. Increasing muscle mass significantly would help maintain your BMR, but this is almost impossible to do while taking in fewer calories than you need every day. Increasing your activity level, especially if you presently are sedentary, does work to a degree, but, over the long run, it's not enough to cancel out the body's response to what it perceives as a mild starvation condition. So, what this means for the typical dieter is that in response to the daily calorie restriction of most diets, the body will adapt and maintain its weight on fewer calories.

The second punch of daily dieting, especially if calorie restriction is severe, lands on the musculature. If you've ever seen anyone who has lost a lot of weight quickly, very often, instead of looking lean and athletic, they look like a smaller version of their overweight selves, basically retaining the same shape they had. This is because, typically, one third of the weight lost in this way is muscle tissue. As if this weren't enough, losing muscle tissue will semi permanently lower your BMR. The only way to restore the BMR, at this point, is to replace the muscle tissue. Rule of thumb: muscle is easier to keep than replace.

By now, you've surely surmised that we are not fans of daily dieting, and certainly not fans of its two basic physiological effects. After all, if your goal is permanent weight loss, why would you use a technique that, after long months of self-discipline, virtually guarantees weight gain because it trains the body to gain fat on fewer calories and hold on to its present fat reserves? Unless you are training for a Sumo Contest, this is pretty much opposite to what you are trying to accomplish.

Monotony Kills Motivation

The second major category of reasons for daily diet failure is, as previously mentioned, a bit more psychological. If you think about prison and ask yourself: how does imprisonment really punish a person? The answer, at least in today's American prisons, is not physical pain, but is really deprivation. Prison deprives the convicted person of all but a few basic options. If you accept that premise, then it is safe to say that, in our society, the most common way we punish serious crime is by taking away most of a criminal's freedom to choose. Oddly enough, most diets require this very same approach, and the success or failure of the diet depends on the ability to symbolically imprison oneself by way of food deprivation. Think about the following scenario, and ask yourself if you haven't been there or somewhere very much like it.

It's a Saturday night in late March. You are on your way to a popular restaurant to visit with old friends you haven't seen in years. As you walk toward your car, an unusually balmy breeze caresses you and makes you think of the sunny beach-days of June that dwell just beyond the horizon. Such sultry weather at this time of the year should be welcome. Instead of putting a smile on your face, though, it actually makes you feel a little disconcerted because you know you will not enjoy those June beach-days unless the bathroom scale says you can. After starting the car, you put it in gear and hope driving will put these thoughts out of your mind.

After a ten-minute drive, the restaurant is in sight. As you near the parking lot, you drive a little slower to give yourself time to gird your willpower against the temptations that lie just a few moments away. You feel yourself becoming a bit flushed as an internal war is beginning to wage within you. When you pull into the parking lot, a valet waves you over and asks if you would like him to park your car. You politely decline and idle away, instead, deciding to park in a far corner of the lot because the walk will burn one or two more carbs or fat grams or whatever your diet has declared fattening. Finally, after finding a suitable spot, you pull in, shut off the engine, and close up the car.

On your self-imposed long walk through the parking lot, doubt begins to tighten its grip on you and you begin to rationalize your anticipated failure. The restaurant now looms closer and closer and your mind searches its card catalog of excuses. Your thought process takes on a life of its own and you begin to think, *'Oh well, so what if I blow it tonight; it's not like I see these friends all the time, or if I blow it tonight, I will simply not eat tomorrow.'* Gradually, the voice in your head begins to take on a soprano then sopranino pitch, screeching excuses at you faster and faster until your thoughts whirl into a jumbled mess. If you could just find something, anything that would let you off the dietary leash for the night, and allow you to forego the self-loathing you always feel after violating your latest diet, you might still be able to enjoy this evening. At the last moment, self-discipline shoulders self-doubt out of the way, and, defiantly, you swear allegiance to your diet and vow to be satisfied by the company of your old friends, if not by the victuals this particular restaurant is known for.

Just before pushing open the front door, you take a deep breath and sigh. Your resolve is now firm, and your thinking is more along the lines of, *'Wouldn't this be a great place to come back to and really enjoy, after I've reached my goal weight.'* Twinges of doubt, again, accompany this bit of introspection. You know this is not the first time you have been on a diet, and you have yet to attain that magical night when you could stop dieting, eat a normal meal and not put five pounds back on. Feeling a bit dejected, you shake off those thoughts, pull open the heavy oaken door, and allow the seductive aromas to drag you in.

As soon as you breach the foyer, you are confronted by the hostess who asks you how many people are in your party. You hesitate as you scan the dining room, finally spotting your old chums who are already seated. You point to their table, explaining that they are your party, and rush off to greet them. As you approach the table, your friends spot you and begin to call out your name. They are obviously in a raucous mood. The affection and camaraderie between you and your friends is palpable. The waitress, who has just arrived to take their drink order, seems to be infected by the good will as she waits patiently for the greetings to be finished with what appears to be a genuine smile on her face.

After the commotion dies down, two of your friends order imported beers and the third asks for a mixed drink with lots of sugar and an umbrella in it. Then it's your turn, and the moment of truth hits you. You are on the amazing "I Can't Eat or Drink Anything That Tastes Good Diet!" Therefore, you cannot have beer, wine, wine coolers, mixed drinks, especially if they have umbrellas in them, orange juice, cola, or anything else with a modicum of flavor. Dejectedly, you order water on the rocks and try to convince yourself that not only is this self-deprivation worth it, but that you really like it.

The waitress returns to deliver the drinks and take your dinner orders just as your friends are complimenting you on your extraordinary self-discipline. Then Sally, who could empty any fast food joint at a sitting and never gain a pound, orders the Pasta Primavera, Cheryl orders the filet mignon with a baked potato and all the trimmings, and Shirley has a burger with fries, "Oh what the hell, put cheese on those thangs." When it's your turn, you smile primly and ask the waitress how many carbohydrates watercress has, and also if it tastes good because if it does, well, you know... You pass the rest of the night in a state of quiet desperation.

This scenario is, of course, a bit of an exaggeration, but it underscores the point that most severely restricted diets eventually become boring. People feel bored, deprived, and even isolated when they have to eat the same food every day, and/or restrict one or more food groups from their lives. These feelings are especially intense when one is on a very low calorie, or elimination diet like the low fat and low or no carbohydrate diets that are so popular today. Anyone who has tried this type of dieting knows the frustration that is inherent in an overly restrictive approach.

At this point, we should note that sometimes for health reasons, it is necessary to avoid certain foods completely; this is not the condition this book is addressing. **Before starting any diet or exercise program, especially if you have a medical problem that requires you to avoid certain foods, you should consult your doctor. This rule applies to everyone.**

I hope I have shed some light on why we contend that approaches to weight loss that require eating less than your body needs, every single day, eventually train your body to hold on to its fat reserves and result in feelings of deprivation, isolation and boredom. A corollary of this is: even if you do manage to make it to your goal weight, as soon as you start eating a more normal amount of calories, the tendency will still be to regain the weight you have lost, because you have not learned how much food you really need, so, driven by hunger, the inclination is to over do it. Like I said before, each time you do this, you lose muscle tissue and regain body fat. Not exactly what most people have in mind when they make the decision to lose weight.

Before you get started, one final scrap of food for thought: you are not a bad person if you eat! You are just responding to a natural survival urge built into you by millions of years of evolution. Guilt has no place in dieting. If you approach dieting objectively and unemotionally, it works better and is less difficult. If you need to feel guilty about something, there are innumerable afternoon television talk shows that can provide plenty of grist for the shame mill.

You could walk to the moon, if you had a chair to sit on
anytime you needed one.

2 | Getting Started

Let's Revisit Gloria And Then Forget Everything You Think You Know About Dieting

Gloria's knee surgery went without a hitch. They only had to repair one ligament and remove part of one cartilage. Within ten days, she found herself in her doctor's office where he told her that she should be able to return to her normal duties in a short time. Given the pain and stiffness in her knee, she questioned the validity of his statement, but said nothing. He then scribbled something on a prescription pad and then, with a sardonic expression, said she would need to start Physical Therapy soon. He recommended a place called The Weighting Room. Gloria chuckled at the name when he first mentioned it. He smiled again and said, "See you in six weeks."

One week later, after dropping the kids off at school, she drove to The Weighting Room, eager to begin her rehab. Upon her arrival, a bubbly medical assistant presented her with the requisite ream of paperwork, now required by insurance companies.

When she was done answering the redundant questions, she handed it back to the bubbly medical assistant, and then sat down to wait to be called back into the gym. From her seat, she could see over a waist-high wall into the workout area. It appeared cheerful with large windows on two sides that provided a lot of natural light, and chrome plated equipment that gave the place a very upbeat, almost futuristic feel. Watching the other people working out while she waited, she experienced a sense of confidence that caused an involuntary smile to brighten her features as she thought she might actually enjoy coming here. Then she met her therapist.

Her name was Danielle, and she would be the first woman since her mother with whom Gloria would have a love/hate relationship, and this after only ten minutes. Danielle stood five-feet nothing and probably weighed 95-pounds. During their first hour together, though, she proved plenty capable, and pitiless as she made Gloria move her knee farther and more frequently than any human should ever have to. Worst of all, throughout the whole ordeal, Danielle wore the most benign smile on her face.

It was during this hell-on-earth that Gloria realized the significance of her doctor's smile when he had handed her the prescription for Physical Therapy. He knew rehabilitating a knee he had just sliced into would not be without its own brand of pain. Even though Gloria knew it was for her own good, she spent much of her time in therapy plotting revenge against her doctor, and all surgeons for that matter. At this point, she didn't plot revenge against Danielle, because she was convinced Danielle was evil and would somehow sense these thoughts and punish her for them.

Dreaming about being able to kick her doctor in the shin on her next visit provided a pleasant diversion while she exercised, but it really wasn't the major motivation for rehabilitating her knee. The far greater motivation was fear. You see, Gloria was starting her college courses in five weeks and the thought of taking courses with people 20-years her junior had her apprehensive enough. She did not need a limp to further underscore the age difference.

Despite the initial pain though, Gloria's rehab went well. Often, while she was enduring set after set of hamstring curls and knee extensions, she would find herself smiling as she thought that it seemed Hugh's "encouragement" had been well-founded. Besides her other exercises, she was quickly introduced to the joy of the stationary bicycle. Within two weeks, she noticed a strange thing. She had lost a pound without sacrificing even one crumb from her normal eating routine.

Gloria mentioned this to Danielle, who said it was common for people to lose a little weight when they first started an exercise program because their bodies were not used to the increased activity. Danielle also added that Gloria's weight would probably stabilize when her body adapted to the exercise regimen. At this, Gloria's mouth drew down into a feigned pout and she said, "But I don't want to adapt."

Danielle laughed and said, "No one does." After another week of exercise, Gloria's weight had indeed stabilized.

One day, while she cranked out revolution after revolution on the stationary bike, a lean, middle-aged woman whisked into the gym, set down a huge purse and enough keys to make any high-rise building superintendent envious on the therapist's desk, and began to peddle the bike next to Gloria's. Immediately after establishing a cadence twice as fast as Gloria's, the woman said hello and introduced herself, extending a well-tanned arm and hand. Her name was Gabi, and she lived up to her name, as she was able to carry on never less than two, and up to five conversations, by Gloria's count, at any one time. While they were peddling, another patient walked by and complimented her on her weight loss. Gabi thanked her and said she still had at least ten more pounds to go. This really got Gloria's attention and she said, "I hope you don't mind my asking, but you don't look like you ever had a weight problem."

Gabi smiled and said, "Oh, that's nice of you to say, but I've lost over fifty pounds since I've been following Danielle's advice."

"Really, how long did that take?"

"A little less than a year, but that was two years ago. For the last year I've been really just maintaining, but now I've decided to lose a little more weight so I can find me a man." She looked at Gloria and winked, then they both giggled like high-schoolers.

When their giddiness subsided, Gloria pressed for more information. "No, seriously, how did you lose the weight?"

Gabi explained that she followed a system where she didn't diet everyday, but on the days she did not diet, she was careful not to overeat. Gloria listened intently to the disjointed explanation and then with a bewildered look asked, "But how do you really know when you have eaten enough, but not overeaten?"

Gabi responded with a very chipper, "Oh, that's easy, you just have to find your BMR and then multiply by your activity level. Then that's the number of calories you can eat and not gain weight. It's really pretty accurate, and when you get it right, you will be surprised that you won't have that always-hungry feeling, like when you're on a regular diet."

Perhaps it was Gabi's abbreviated explanation, or the fact that her Boston accent precluded her from pronouncing the letter R -which meant BMR came out BMAHHHH- but Gloria felt more confused after the explanation than before. She pressed on, "Did you say Danielle helped you with this?"

"Oh yes, she figured out my calories and walked me through the system for a few weeks."

Gloria's eyes narrowed as she thought, *'That little torturer has been holding out on me.'* When her time on the stationary cycle was up, Gloria corralled Danielle and asked her to explain the system to her. Danielle gave Gabi a little side-glance and then smiled resignedly before saying that she did not have the time that day to fully explain it. Gloria's frown told Danielle that she wasn't really happy with that response, so she then asked Gloria if her weight had been relatively stable for the last few months. Before Gloria could answer, another patient bellowed for Danielle from one of the treatment rooms. Danielle held up her index finger in a wait-a-minute gesture and told Gloria to hold the thought. When Danielle returned from emergency pillow repositioning, Gloria said her weight had been fairly stable, with the exception of the recent one-pound weight loss, for the last year. Danielle nodded, almost solemnly, and told her to simply cut whatever portions she had been eating in half for three days each week. Gloria shook her head and said, "Which three days?"

Danielle answered, "Any three days in a given week, and they don't have to be bunched together. In fact, they don't even have to be the same ones every week."

Gloria shot back, "That just sounds too simple."

Danielle retorted, "You know it's a funny thing about reality, often the simplest answer is the right one."

Gloria thought about this for a minute and said, "What's Gabi talking about with the BMR and the activity level?"

"That's all part of it, but I don't have time to give you a good explanation today." Gloria's look of confusion and desperation seemed to strike a sympathetic chord in Danielle and she said, "Tell you what, since getting fitter and losing weight is really integral to your knee rehab, we'll set aside some time in the next few weeks to really go over it. Meanwhile, just start by cutting your calories in half on three days per week."

On her drive home, a ray of hope began to push back the shadows of doubt, as Gloria thought, *'This is really a different way to do this.'* A cautious smile then brightened her features as she reflected, *'This could really work for me.'* She started her new approach the next day.

Over the next three weeks Gloria lost four pounds. On the days when she ate her full calorie complement, she felt certain that there was no way that this could result in a net weight loss, but each week, after she saw a lower weight on the bathroom scale, she felt her skepticism crumble just a little more. The holiday season came and went and Gloria discovered that she had not gained any weight during that time, but she had not lost any either. She wasn't sure why, but she suspected that she might have eaten more on her full calorie days than she intended. She would try to get some answers when she resumed therapy after the holidays.

On the third day of January, Gloria awoke to find the world outside was covered by a pristine mantle of snow. She was scheduled for rehab that day and she wondered if they would even be open. Before she got too far into her morning routine, she checked her answering machine, and seeing no blinking red light, she concluded that they had not called to cancel. Gloria wanted to get in every session she could to minimize her gimp before school started in a little over two weeks. Just to be on the safe side though, she called to confirm and sure enough, they were having hours.

Upon arriving, she shook off the cold, and with only a slight limp, walked back into the unusually quiet gym. Though it was just after 8:00 A.M., Gabi was already there and had her bike up to what appeared to be a sixty-miles-per-hour pace. Gloria nodded at Gabi as she mounted the bike next to hers. Gabi said a quick, "Hi," before returning to her argument with two staff members and another patient regarding their interpretations of the most recent professional football games.

When Gloria's twenty-five-minute ride was done, she stepped off her bike and grabbed a towel from a shelf next to the bikes and wiped the sweat from her face. Gabi was still arguing and peddling, and appeared as fresh as Lance Armstrong on the first day of the Tour de France.

After a short break, Gloria then meandered over to the weight rack and pulled two red ten-pound strap weights down from their hooks. She then sat down on one of the mat tables to strap them to her ankles in preparation for her leg exercises. Just as she was starting her exercises, Danielle appeared from one of the treatment rooms, sat down on the table next to Gloria and asked how her knee was feeling. Gloria saw her chance and said that although her knee was fine, she had questions about the diet Danielle had recommended. Danielle looked around the empty gym, laughed, and agreed that this might be their only chance to give a semi-full explanation of the approach.

As Gloria pumped iron, Danielle first explained why traditional diets had failed Gloria in the past. This explanation gave her a good idea of what BMR meant, what affected it, and why traditional daily dieting lowered it. Finally, Danielle calculated Gloria's BMR and multiplied it by the correct activity factor to give her a good approximation of her daily and then weekly caloric need.

Although it was a lot to digest in a short period of time, Gloria absorbed it like a sponge because it agreed with her past experiences with dieting, and because it seemed to offer a truly different, and logical approach.

After Danielle laid the groundwork for the system, Gloria had a few questions. "Danielle, that all sounds logical, but why can't I just stay on the program I'm on now? It's so simple to just cut my portions in half, rather than actually count calories."

"Didn't you say that you didn't lose any weight over the holidays?"

"Well, yes," Gloria admitted.

"Did you cut your portions in half on at least three days?"

"Yes, and I was very proud of myself, but I think I see where you're going with this. You think I made up for it on the full-calorie days."

"Or maybe your light days weren't as light as you thought. Don't get me wrong, there are people who innately have a good sense of this, but for most of us, an objective guide, or compass if you will, is necessary. Otherwise, over time, most people have a tendency to eat more on their full calorie days because they are naturally a little hungry after the light days, and the tendency is for the body to prod you into consuming the missing calories. In other words, you have to learn when enough is enough."

"Oh, so that means I'll have to count calories forever?"

"Not necessarily, it just takes time to learn when enough is enough. Also, when you follow this system for a while, your stomach will tend to shrink, which will make the feeling of fullness happen with fewer calories, and become a better gauge of whether or not you have eaten enough."

"So, if you've been overeating a lot and stretching your stomach, not feeling full does not necessarily mean you should eat more."

"That's right, when you eat, your blood sugar level rises to tell the brain when to stop eating. This is not the same as feeling full. Let me give you a little rule of thumb. If you use this approach correctly, by the second full-calorie day, you shouldn't have the chronic hunger that never seems to be satisfied, even right after meals, when you're on a traditional diet." Gloria smiled, in spite of herself at this, and Danielle chided, "Aha, I see you know what I mean. Practically anyone who has ever dieted on an everyday basis for any amount of time knows that feeling."

Gloria nodded as she remembered exactly what Danielle was talking about. Many systems she had tried left her feeling exactly that way.

Nothing was worse than that unrelenting feeling of hunger that haunted you without respite, even after you had eaten whatever the diet allowed for a given meal. In retrospect, she could see that this was the downfall of all her other weight loss attempts. "So then, you are saying that a person is not dieting on the full calorie days?"

"That's exactly right, not dieting but not overeating."

"So then a person is only dieting on the low calorie days?"

"Yes."

"Then why not do six low calorie days each week? I mean, if a person could just force themselves to deal with the hunger, wouldn't that be quicker?"

"Isn't that very close to what you've tried in the past, and isn't that what has always failed in the long run?" Danielle raised her eyebrows in a look of mock disapproval and Gloria could only sheepishly grin.

"So what you're saying is that each week, a person should go on a mini-diet and then maintain, and then diet and then maintain and so on. Sort of like dividing the big job of losing weight into small tasks and then accomplish each one, one at a time."

"Bingo," Danielle said, as she nodded affirmatively, but before she could expound on this, a bell rang in one of the treatment rooms and she had to excuse herself.

By now you might think that Danielle is trying to stuff a ten-pound explanation into a five-pound bag. It's not that she wants to give Gloria short shrift, but anyone who has been to a busy rehab center knows the therapists have roughly negative three seconds to spend with each patient. Since we in "book land" have no such constraints, we can afford to break the system down and make sure everybody is on the same page, especially with regard to some common and not-so-common definitions.

Later on, we will look in on Gloria to see exactly how she handled those first days of her new life, but for now, pay attention because there is no way that Danielle is going to have the time to tell you all this in one sitting.

Let's Get This Kaiser Rolling

Before beginning this approach, you must know two important numbers. They are the number of calories per day, and the number of calories per week it takes for you to maintain your present body weight. For the purposes of this book, we will call these your <u>Daily Caloric Need (DCN), and Weekly Caloric Need (WCN)</u>. Daily caloric need is not the same as basal metabolic rate (<u>BMR</u>). Your DCN is your BMR plus the calories burned by your daily activities. This includes calories burned as a result of your job duties, activities at home, and any exercise program in which you may be involved. To calculate your WCN, you will simply take your DCN and multiply by seven. The interplay between these two numbers is the heart and soul of this approach, and I hope to convey a good understanding of this concept by the end of this chapter.

Before we discuss calculating your DCN, we need to make a few things clear about activity. The first is that all activity, or movement, burns calories, and the second is that the number of calories a given activity uses is different for each person. These differences are caused by body size, amount of muscle and genetics.

For example, a 250-pound football player will burn more calories hanging clothes for a half-hour than a 90-pound woman performing the same task. Because this is such a low intensity activity, you might think body size wouldn't matter, but it is a basic law of physics that to move a larger object the same distance requires more energy.

If the 90-pound woman has a body fat percentage of 40 percent, meaning 40 percent of her weight is composed of fat; she will always burn fewer calories for any given activity than a 90-pound woman who has 20 percent of her weight as body fat. This is because muscle burns more calories than fat, even when at rest, and the woman with the lower body fat has a greater amount of muscle tissue.

Finally, there is the dreaded, uncontrollable, stuck-with-what-you-got, genetic background. We all know people who can eat whatever they want and never gain an ounce, or people who hear somebody else talk about a picture of a piece of cheesecake and gain five pounds. Thankfully, most of us fall somewhere in the middle.

Now we can talk about determining your daily caloric need (DCN). There are two ways you can use to calculate this. The first way is to keep a diary of everything you eat for a week and then, with the help of a good calorie counter, (available in bookstores, or the Internet) simply add up the calories. This will give you a pretty good idea of your WCN. To find your average DCN, you would simply divide your WCN by seven. Remember, this must be done during a week in which your weight remains unchanged. If you are diligent and really keep track of the weights and amounts of the foods eaten, this can be fairly accurate. The second and more typical way we recommend to calculate DCN is to first use the "Harris Benedict

Formula," [1] which uses your age, height, sex, and weight, to calculate your BMR.

For women, the formula is:
BMR = 655 + (4.36 X weight in pounds) + (4.57 X height in inches)- (4.7 X age in years)

For men, the formula is:
BMR = 66 + (6.22 X weight in pounds) + (12.7 X height in inches) - (6.8 X age in years)

☺ Incidentally, if you're not comfortable with the math, there is a table at the back of the book where you can simply look up your BMR.

After you have calculated your BMR, you simply multiply by the applicable activity multiplier listed below. The same multipliers are used for both men and women.
   -If you are Sedentary (little or no exercise)
   Calorie-Calculation = BMR X 1.2
   -If you are Lightly Active (light exercise/sports 1-3
   days/week) Calorie-Calculation = BMR X 1.375
   -If you are Moderately Active (moderate exercise/sports 3-5
   days/week) Calorie-Calculation = BMR X 1.55
   -If you are Very Active (hard exercise/sports 6-7
   days/week) Calorie-Calculation = BMR X 1.725
   -If you are Extra Active (very hard daily exercise/sports &
   physical job or 2X day training) Calorie-Calculation = BMR
   X 1.9

Who would like an example? I know I like examples. Oh, what the heck, here's an example. Let's say Jane is a 45-year-old woman who weighs 140 pounds and is 66 inches tall. She has an administrative job that requires some walking; she works out three days per week, and she likes to play tennis on the weekend. Her calculation would go like this:⇒⇒⇒⇒⇒

---

[1] Julia Layton. *"How Calories Work"*. October 26, 2000 http://health.howstuffworks.com/calorie.htm (January 04, 2008)

4.36 x 140 (her weight in pounds) = <u>610.4</u>   Let's call this her "weight product."

4.57 x 66 (her height in inches) = <u>301.6</u>   Let's call this her "height product."

4.70 x 45 (her age in years) = <u>211.5</u> Let's call this her "age product."

Now add the "weight product" to the "height product" and add 655 to that number, and then subtract the "age product" from that mess. In Jane's case it looks like:

655 + 610 (weight product) + 301.6 (height product) – 211.5 (age product) = BMR 1355, or 655 + 610 + 301.6 - 211.5 = 1355

Now that we know her BMR is 1355, we simply multiply by the appropriate number, which, based on her activity level, is 1.55. This calculates her DCN at a little over 2100 calories per day.

This formula is fairly accurate for most people; however, if you have a very high level of body fat, it may overestimate the number of calories you need to maintain your body weight. If you have very little body fat, i.e., you are very lean, it may underestimate the number of calories you need to maintain your bodyweight. In other words, a 250-pound body builder with eight percent body fat needs more calories than a 250-pound couch potato with 28 percent body fat. This is because, you already know the answer, muscle cells require much more energy to remain alive than fat cells. For most people, a good rule of thumb is: if you need to lose more than 20 percent of your present body weight, then you might want to use a weight about halfway between your present weight and your goal weight, instead of your present weight, to calculate your DCN. If you need to lose less than 20 percent of your body weight, then you can get away with using your present weight to calculate your DCN. Remember, this DCN number is just to get you in the game. It can and probably will be fine-tuned up or down as you see how your weight responds. Again, dieting will be defined as eating less than your DCN.

If you are still unsure of how to do this, use the table at the back of this book or one of the many Internet websites that will calculate this for free. If you use this formula, and you are honest about your activity level, it should provide you with a good caloric starting point.

A great way to test the validity of your DCN calculation is to eat your DCN for seven days before starting to diet. If your weight stays the same, and your hunger is satisfied after you eat, i.e., you are not chronically hungry between meals, then you are probably correct in your calculation. In fact, if you have been habitually dieting, or have been stuck at a plateau, it is not a bad idea to sort of jump-start your BMR by eating your full DCN for at least a week before starting this weight loss system.

After calculating this number, many people are pleasantly surprised at the number of calories they can eat while still maintaining their weight. Chronic dieters usually respond with cautious skepticism and say something like, "I could never eat that much," or, "If I ate that much, I'd be as big as a house!" This thinking is the perfectly logical conclusion of the aforementioned *"dieting, hitting a plateau and then more severely dieting to the next plateau,"* syndrome. Fortunately, it is the wrong conclusion and just a remnant of their experience with <u>daily</u> dieting, and the ever-plummeting BMR that it creates.

OK, so you've calculated your DCN. Now, what can you do with it? Well, you could use it to maintain your bodyweight if you wanted to, and eventually you will, but that's not why you bought this book. You bought it to lose weight! So, let's start by talking about that in the four simple rules outlined below, but, before you read them, I would like you to ponder the power of knowing your DCN. Simply stated, once you reach your goal weight, if you know your correct DCN, there's no reason for you to ever regain weight. That statement will have more significance as we go on. Incidentally, these four rules will ultimately be incorporated into a broader approach that includes weight maintenance as well as weight loss. Now, let's look at those four rules for beginning weight loss.

1- **You will not eat <u>more</u> than your DCN**. For sake of clarity, we will refer to days on which you eat your full DCN as "full-days."

2- **You will <u>not</u> restrict your caloric intake below your DCN more than four days per week, i.e., you will not diet more than four days per week**. So, if your DCN is 2200 calories per day, during a typical week, you will eat some number of calories less than that on no more than four out of seven days. We say no more than four because for many people, eating less than their DCN will only be necessary on three or fewer days. Days on which you eat less than your DCN will be referred to as "light-days."

3- Since we are looking for long-term body fat loss, you should **structure your light-days so that at the end of the week, you have subtracted 3500 calories from your WCN**. This will produce a one-pound per week weight loss. This is a general rule of thumb that applies to most of us, and will be explained further in the next section.

4- **Do some form of regular exercise to maintain muscle mass**. This is paramount to maintaining your normal BMR (basal metabolic rate) and critical to allowing you to eat normally when the weight loss portion of this program is over.

Although four days is the recommended limit for light-days, on very rare occasions, we will employ five light-days for someone who is at the "small" end of the Bell Curve and bent on achieving a one-pound per week weight loss, or to help someone break through a stubborn plateau. We still subtract 3500 calories from the WCN, but over five days instead of three or four. If you do this, we would recommend using it only as a last resort, and for no more than one month, as it is perilously close to daily dieting, and gives the body little time to adjust during the two full-DCN days.

Sounds simple, and it can be, but within this simple framework resides a tremendous amount of flexibility for the dieter. This flexibility and the part-time nature of this program are the two main reasons why the "Part-Time Diet Approach" requires minimal will power, especially compared to more traditional forms of daily dieting. This will become clearer as you see how the plan is actually executed.

Implementing The Plan

Nutritionists agree that a one-pound per week weight loss is both healthy and sustainable. Whether one pound per week is doable for you depends on your body size, muscle mass and activity level. A five-foot tall woman whose weight should be 100 pounds and is currently 105 pounds may not be able to lose a pound per week, because it amounts to a greater percentage of her body weight than a woman whose body weight may be 125 pounds or greater. By this same logic, a man who weighs 300 pounds or more can lose even more than a pound per week, but the vast majority of us fall into the pound per week range.

In order to lose a pound per week, you need to remove 3500 calories from your WCN. A "daily diet" approach might be to simply remove 500 calories per day from your diet to produce a one-pound per week weight loss. As mentioned before, this daily dieting eventually results in the body lowering its need for calories. "The Part-Time Diet Approach" would have you concentrate the 3500-calorie deficit into three or four days, and allow you to eat your full DCN the other days. The reason we do it this way is that eating different amounts of food on different days seems to keep the body "confused," and thwarts the tendency to lower its calorie needs in response to what it perceives as a starvation event. In other words, by dieting for just a few days and then eating your full DCN, the next three or four days, you never give the body time to adjust its calorie need down to meet the new caloric intake. Remember, when you eat your full DCN, you are not dieting.

The possible combinations with this way of thinking are almost limitless. Let's just say you are an average-sized, fairly active female, and your DCN is 2200. A simple combination you could use is to just cut your calories in half three days per week. Two thousand two hundred divided by two is 1100, so on your light-days, you would be eating 1100 calories less than you need to maintain your weight. If you do this on any three days per week, it will give you a 3300-calorie deficit for that week. You would only need a 200-calorie deficit on one of the other days, to make a 3500-calorie deficit for the week. To see how this might work, check out the table below.

	Mon	Tues	Wed	Thur	Fri	Sat	Sun
DCN	2200	2200	2200	2200	2200	2200	2200
Cals Eaten	1100	1100	1100	2000	2200	2200	2200
Deficit	1100	1100	1100	200	0	0	0
Adding the deficit row, we get a shortage for the week of 3500.							

So, according to this table, if you eat 1100 calories on Monday, Tuesday, and Wednesday, and on Thursday eat 2000, you will have created a 3500-calorie deficit for the week by dieting only four days. On Friday, Saturday and Sunday, you must eat 2200 calories: no more or less. If you had decided you really wanted to diet only three days out of the week, you could have created that last little 200 calorie deficit by just walking an extra five minutes per day throughout the week. At the risk of being repetitive, this means most people can achieve a one-half to one-pound per week weight loss by dieting three days per week. Since the number of calories on the light-days does not have to be the same, you could also do two days at 1100 and two days at 1500, and then three days at 2200. In this case, you would create a 3600-calorie shortage for the week by dieting four, less-restrictive, days.

See the table below.

	Mon	Tues	Wed	Thur	Fri	Sat	Sun
DCN	2200	2200	2200	2200	2200	2200	2200
Cals Eaten	1100	1500	1500	1100	2200	2200	2200
Deficit	1100	700	700	1100	0	0	0
Total calorie deficit or shortage for the week is 3600.							

To reiterate, you would not diet more than four days in any given week, and you would not eat more than your DCN, which, in this case, would be 2200.

It should be starting to become apparent that this approach allows for an almost infinite number of choices. You can vary the days on which you diet, you can vary the number of calories you eat, you can vary the amount of exercise you do, and, of course, you can vary the actual foods you eat. With this approach, no food is "fattening", but some foods cost more. Think of a calorie checking account in which you, using the example above, deposit 15400 (2200 X 7) calories per week. The penalty for overdrawing on your account by eating too many calories is weight gain. Remember, this is not like the government that can spend like there is no tomorrow. So, if you want cheesecake after dinner, it will cost you, but you CAN have it.

Paradoxically, some of the main advantages of this approach lie in what it does NOT require you to do. It does not require you to eat only certain foods, in fact, it will work better if you eat meals that borrow from a wide range of food groups rather than, let's say, a strict chocolate bar and French fry regimen. As previously stated, it also does not require you to diet every day; in fact, even the mildly attentive reader knows, "The Part-Time Diet Approach" prohibits ever-day dieting. A corollary of that idea is that there is no rigid system that dictates exactly what days you will diet, or how much you will eat; there is only a framework of rules that you are free to apply according to your lifestyle. If this is still unclear, don't worry; there will be examples and more detail in the upcoming chapters.

If you are a devotee of some other diet plan, you can use this approach to enhance the plan you are already on, or, perhaps, use it to break through a sticking point. It could be as simple as eating whatever your diet calls for, but cutting your normal amounts by half or a third, a few days per week.

Remember, this approach works precisely because your daily food intake varies. Reversing the typical dieting process, it makes food intake a moving target that challenges the body to adapt to it instead of you adapting your intake to the ever-decreasing BMR.

One of the most important implications of this fact is that, with the right type of exercise, when you reach your goal weight, you will have lost little or no muscle tissue, so your BMR will be largely preserved. That means you will not have to constantly starve yourself to maintain your new weight. Once you become sensitive to your daily caloric need, you won't ever have to be overweight again.

What To Expect

Let's assume you have decided to use the first approach mentioned above where you will simply eat half of your DCN three days per week and your full DCN four days per week. Although losing one pound per week is thought to be the best way to attain long-term weight loss, during the first week, it is not uncommon to lose two to four pounds. Probably two out of the four pounds will be water weight, but even this is not bad because it will make clothes fit better and, if you have hypertension or congestive heart failure, losing what amounts to a little more than a quart of excess fluid will almost certainly improve these conditions.

For most people, within a few weeks, weight loss will stabilize to roughly a pound per week. Again, what days you pick to diet is entirely up to you. This author's preference is to string them together. You may prefer to spread them out for whatever reason. Either way works just as well. As mentioned above, you don't need to use the same days every week either, in fact, varying the days is yet another way to keep the body guessing. So, if you find you must work an unusually long shift on a planned light-day, you can simply make it a full-day and make some other day your light-day.

Now, what about hunger? Well, let's say you've decided to follow a schedule that calls for light-days on Monday, Tuesday and Wednesday. By Wednesday, you will be hungry, but, starting Thursday, you can look forward to eating your full DCN for four days. If you are correct in your DCN calculation, by Friday, you will feel like you are not even dieting. By Sunday, you will be rested and ready to start the next "light-day" cycle. Do you remember the lady in the previous chapter who met with her friends in the restaurant? Imagine how different that scenario would have been if she was following this program. She could have used a full DCN day and actually eaten a real meal, while still remaining true to her weight loss program. This is the power of this type of approach. ⇒⇒⇒⇒⇒⇒⇒⇒

Tips For Getting Through The Light-Days

Since the light days will obviously be the hardest to stick to, I would like to offer you a few tips I have learned over the years from my as well as other's experiences.

> - Plan meals, especially in the beginning. This can be as simple as just taking your lunch to work.
> - High fiber carbohydrate sources like fruits, vegetables, some types of cereal, nuts, and whole-grain breads can stabilize blood sugar. This helps control hunger and, because of the fiber content, these foods can make one feel fuller on fewer calories.
> - Eat slowly. It can take twenty minutes or more for your blood sugar to rise to the point where your hypothalamus (an area in the brain that detects sugar levels in the blood among other things) tells you you're not hungry any more.
> - Be realistic. It has been our experience that trying to eat less than 1000 calories per day for four days per week is very difficult for any adult, regardless of their size. However, in some people, two or three days per week may be manageable, it really depends on your DCN.
> - Sleep! For sufferers of insomnia, this can be tough, but good sleep will definitely help you remain true to your caloric limits.
> - Vary Foods. This can be instrumental in preventing that deprived feeling most dieters go through. If you find yourself in a food rut, eating the same things day after day, try checking out your local supermarket. Most things are labeled and, especially here in America, we are blessed with almost unlimited variety.
> - Drink hot liquids before meals. Drinking hot liquids often produces a feeling of fullness.
> - Eat protein. Protein can take longer to leave the stomach and decrease hunger between meals.
> - Eat something small, like a piece of fruit, 20 minutes before a meal. This really helps squelch the tendency to overeat.
> - Get a diet partner. This can really help when you want to split large portions. I have actually known like-minded dieting friends who set aside one day a month to meet up and try out new dishes. The fact that they could split the cuisine made their food choices almost limitless.

> ➢ Unless you're a veteran calorie counter, avoid buffets or unfamiliar situations, at least in the beginning, and especially on light-days.
> ➢ Some restaurants tend to give large portions to make you feel like you've gotten more for your money. Rather than petition the Congress to write new laws to protect us from this practice, why not just use the old doggie bag routine. Taking food home and eating it on some other day, instead of trying to eat more than you need in one sitting, is great for the waistline. In addition, you have also gotten two meals for the price of one, and that's good for the wallet. Sounds like a win-win to us. This is almost like becoming your own dieting partner.
> ➢ Stay busy. If you sit around and think about food, you will find reasons to eat. If your mind is focused on other things, you will be surprised at how long you can go without eating. Everybody has a friend that will occasionally say, "Oh, I just forgot to eat today." Instead of allowing this to bring out, perfectly reasonable and understandable, homicidal tendencies in us, we should just learn a lesson from this, which is: if you stay busy, you will be less likely to dwell on your own, often exaggerated, sense of hunger.

Dealing With Plateaus

Anyone who has tried to lose a significant amount of weight knows what a plateau is with respect to dieting. For our purposes, we will define it as two consecutive weeks with no weight loss. It has been my experience that, occasionally, you can go a week and do everything correctly and still end up with the scale reading the same or higher. If this happens to you, don't panic. It does not necessarily mean you have gained body fat or even plateaued. It is, more often than not, water weight from some extra salt, or carbs in the diet, or bad timing for the weigh-in relative to the last time you used the bathroom.

However, if after two weeks, you have not lost any weight, then you have probably reached the, aforementioned, dreaded plateau. Unfortunately, plateaus are a fact of life in any diet program. The difference in how this approach handles them, though, may pleasantly surprise the veteran dieter. With this approach, the answer is not to further reduce calories or increase time in the gym. The way The Part-Time Diet Approach recommends you deal with plateaus is to do something different. By different, I mean changing the number of calories you eat on your light-days, or changing your activities. Allow me to repeat, the answer is <u>NOT</u> to further decrease your calories or increase exercise intensity or activity time. For example, if you're dieting three days, you might just reshuffle your calories, i.e., eat more on your light-days, but use four light-days instead of three. Remember, the number of calories on the light-days does not have to be the same, so, to use the example from above, if three days at 1100 calories loses its effectiveness, four days at 1325 or two at 1100 and two at 1500 will work. Any combination will work as long as the four basic rules are followed.

After some time, especially with people who have a lot of weight to lose, no amount of shuffling may seem to push you over the next precipice. The answer to this conundrum is even more counterintuitive. In order to resume weight loss, you must eat your full DCN for one week. That is: to use the previous example, 2200 calories per day for seven days. Most people are surprised that when they do this, not only do they not gain a lot of weight back, but they usually blow right through the plateau when they resume the diet. When you use this tactic, you may or may not see a pound or two increase on the scale at the weekly weigh-in during the week you eat your full DCN. If you do, it's OK and only reflects a little fluid retention because you're eating a little more.

Let's Slap The Wrap On This Chunk Of Cheese

You now have all the basic tools to execute the dietary portion of this approach. First, you find your BMR; you can use the previously described formula or the table in the back of this book. Then you find your DCN (BMR plus activities), and then multiply by seven to calculate your WCN. Remember, if you are careful, you can also use the calorie counting method to determine your DCN and WCN, or simply go to my website (http://www.parttimediet.com), which has a calculator that will, after asking you some probing questions like height, weight, age and gender, simply give you your number. Don't get too obsessive over these numbers; these methods of determining your BMR, DCN, and WCN are used only to give you a starting point. You can fine-tune your calorie intake as you go.

Next, subtract some number of calories from your WCN –3500 equals one pound- and decide which days will be your full and light-days, and how many calories you will subtract on the light-days to achieve the weekly deficit you have chosen. These days are not cast in stone and can change from week to week. Don't neglect eating on the full-days. This is critical to getting through the light-days. The ultimate success of this plan depends on not eating less than your DCN every day. If you do eat less than your DCN every day, you will eventually encounter all the problems inherent in the "diet-every-day" type of approach.

Remember, most of us have not gotten fat overnight, or by continually gorging ourselves. It is usually a gradual accumulation of 100 or 200 calories, a few days a week, until one day we look at our reflection and exclaim, "Who put this funhouse mirror in my bathroom?" The best way to dig yourself out is the way you dug yourself in: slowly, so you will -let's say it again- maintain your skeletal muscle. Muscle tissue is a major contributing factor to your BMR and must be maintained for long-term weight loss. Diets that promise quick weight loss largely ignore this and, without superhuman willpower, will eventually fail. Some of you might be thinking, *'OK fine, I don't have to diet every day, but I still have to count calories; I hate counting calories. I would rather go to a daily IRS audit than count calories.'* In the next chapter, we will see how Gloria handles this, and give you some ammunition to make this formerly onerous task easier. You will also be shown the endless culinary options available to you when you become familiar with the common caloric values that exist within families of foods. Once you see these patterns, IRS audits and the act of counting calories can be put back into their proper perspective.

Think Checking Account

On this day, of all days, Gloria had gotten held up at work, so now she had only one hour to shower, dress and get to her first college class in twenty years. After dressing, she examined herself for fit and finish in her dresser mirror. Her younger co-workers had assured her that jeans and a sweater would be perfectly appropriate wear for night school, so she had bought new blue jeans and a mauve knit cotton sweater. Everything fit well, and she smiled at her reflection. The weight-loss plan and the exercise had already begun to pay visible dividends, and she felt optimistic and even downright youthful.

Another payoff of the last six weeks' diligence was a near perfect gait on level ground. She still had some problems with stairs, though. Specifically, if she went up more than two flights at a time, her knee would ache for a while, but this too was resolving, albeit slowly. Danielle had told her that as she got closer to full function, the last few degrees of movement and strength would take the longest, so Gloria was not discouraged.

The college Gloria had chosen was located just outside Philadelphia. It was constructed in the late 1800s in what the brochures called a "Romanesque" style. True to this architectural bent, the outer walls were constructed of stone, and gave the appearance of being very thick, like one would see in a medieval castle. Gloria had liked the feel of the place when she came here for open house, almost five months ago. She also liked the classrooms, which reminded her, for all the world, of her elementary school. They had real blackboards with built-in wooden chalk ledges, and six-foot tall windows in the outer bulkheads that actually opened. An unfortunate attribute of these windows was that in a typical three-hour class, they leaked enough air to fill the "Underdog Balloon" at Macy's® Thanksgiving Day Parade. Barely offsetting this seepage, cast iron radiators, running under the windows and slopped with the same beige paint as the walls, would hiss, and bang, and groan during the winter months, while hellishly hot steam coursed through them.

The irony of teaching the latest in high tech education in classrooms that felt like time capsules from the Eisenhower era was not lost on her. This "quaintness" though, presented other problems besides heating and cooling. Keeping 30 new computers running and properly communicating with each other, and their designated server, in a classroom whose electrical system was originally designed to run a few light bulbs presented many ongoing "issues" for the school's maintenance department, issues, which often necessitated the moving of classes. For instance, classes originally scheduled for room 125 to room 417.

Traffic on the way to the college was worse than she had expected, so Gloria arrived a little later than she would have liked. This did not really concern her until she read the handwritten, notebook-paper sign on the door to room 125, proclaiming relocation of her first class. Since she already knew the elevator's reputation for "speed" she decided to risk climbing the stairs. As she toughed out the four flights, she thought, '*The universe has a sense of humor.*' Despite all her good intentions and effort, she would limp into the first class she had attended in twenty years. This was not what bothered her most though. She felt like the stair-climb was a metaphor for what she was sure was the daunting task of learning ahead. To her, it felt like stepping back in time to finish unfinished business.

When she reached the fourth-floor landing, she stopped a moment, gave herself a good symbolic shaking, and forced her mind to focus on the positive aspect of this experience, namely, stepping into the next chapter in her life. After a short walk down the hallway, she was there.

Room 417 was brightly lit by what seemed to be a hundred fluorescent light bulbs, and populated by many examples of the infamous desk chair:

basically a small hard chair with a writing surface mounted to one side. Her back began to ache just looking at them.

Gloria reflexively migrated to a seat in one of the middle rows. As she squeezed past some of the other students who were milling around waiting for class to begin, two things hit her. The first was that no one noticed her or her limp. She would have been disappointed if she weren't so relieved. The other thing she noticed was that the percentage of twenty-somethings was probably closer to 30 percent, versus the 90-percent she had expected. Gloria, it appeared, was in the chronological majority. She smiled as she settled in for her first three-hour class.

January soon fell into February, which morphed into March. Gloria found that she had little time to worry about such trivial issues as a slight limp, or her age. Her new academic pursuit kept her plenty busy. Over the weeks though, she slowly got to know her fellow students through trips to the snack room, and the occasional study group conducted in whatever empty classroom happened to be available. Sometimes, after she would contribute something to the group, her mind would wander back to that first night, and she would smile at how far she had come.

During this time, people began to comment on her continuing weight loss, and soon, almost every trip to the snack room featured a reluctant Gloria explaining the program in a piecemeal fashion to someone wanting to lose weight for the approaching summer. One night, Gloria was standing in front of the vending machine from which she had just bought a pack of peanut butter crackers. As she perused the label for the number of calories, she could feel the presence of someone looking over her shoulder.

She turned to see one of her classmates evidently trying to read the label also. She knew him, but only cursorily. His name was Phil. He was a tall, heavyset man who appeared to be in his early forties. Gloria liked his sense of humor in class, but during their forays to the snack room, he mostly stayed to himself. She sensed this attempt to communicate with her was a great effort for him, so she held the crackers closer to him. His voice quavered a little as he said, "HMMM, 200 calories in those. I guess you're off your diet." Gloria furrowed her brow in a look of mock anger. This caused a wide-eyed look of panic to cross his face and he said, "Oh I don't mean you look like it, but I mean, isn't 200 calories fattening?"

Gloria smiled a wry smile and said, "Nothing is fattening, and everything is fattening."

Phil looked at her, puzzled, and said, "What?"

She laughed, still not used to being in the role of "diet educator", and said, "If your body needs those calories, they are not fattening, if it doesn't need them, then they are."

He thought about that for a second and said, "You have to admit though, calorie counting is a royal pain."

She wasn't sure if he was just making an awkward attempt at small talk, or if he was challenging her little system. Either way, she didn't feel like defending the program. After all, she was a still a novice at it herself, and it worked for her and that was really all that mattered. She turned and faced him and said, "Well then, this might not be for you. I mean, no system will work without at least some discipline."

Phil looked stung as he retorted, "Well, it's just that I don't know how people do it, counting every calorie and watching every crumb."

"No one said you had to that." Pausing for a moment to gather her thoughts, she continued, "You know, I used to be just like you. I've tried counting calories before and failed, so I gave up. It was by sheer chance that I was introduced to this technique."

"What technique? Isn't losing weight simply a matter of eating less?"

Despite Gloria's reluctance to defend her method, she found herself doing just that when she answered his interrogatory with a question of her own, "Have you ever been on a diet where you, to use your words, simply ate less?"

"Sure, I guess."

"I hope you're not offended by this question, but you did bring up this subject."

"Shoot."

"Well, do you feel your efforts were successful?"

"If you mean, do I think I am overweight now, the answer is yes." Then growing more flustered, he answered a question he wasn't even asked, "But that's because I lost focus and stopped watching what I ate."

"Is it?"

"Well, what do you think it is?"

"When you say you ate less, Phil, it is Phil, isn't it?" She knew his name, but she decided to tweak him because she did not like the growing irritation in his voice. "The logical question is less than what?"

"Well," he thought for a second. "Less than normal. I guess eating less in one way or another is the basis for every diet I've ever tried."

"Less than normal? But you still feel, you're overwei..., umm you still want to lose weight?"

"It's OK, you can say overweight, and the answer is yes, I do want to lose weight."

Gloria felt a little petty for her slip of the tongue, but didn't quite feel her indiscretion met the threshold for an apology, so she just continued, "Then would you agree that just 'eating a little less than normal,' every day has not really worked long-term?"

Phil started to look like a six-year old who had just been chastised by his mom, and sounded almost petulant when he said, "So what's so special about this technique?"

Gloria could not help rolling her eyes before she said, "If you really want to know, I'll tell you how I got started. From there, you're on your own." She paused for a moment and could see he looked a little hurt. Feeling bad, she said, "I'm sorry if that sounds harsh. It's just that it becomes tiring when person after person asks about the system, and before I'm even done with a brief outline, they are shaking their heads, and I can see they're dismissing it before I even finish." Just then, a panicked look crossed Phil's face as he realized he was shaking his head. She picked up on it and began to smile, "It's OK Phil, you were shaking your head yes."

Just then, she looked around and realized they were standing in an abandoned snack room. "Phil, I believe we need to get back to class; if you want, we can pick this up some other time?"

He surprised her when he said, "How about after class? We can stop at the 'Trolley Stop' for a beer."

The color drained from her face, and before she could regain her poise, she stammered, "Umm, I'm still married, and besides, my kids are expecting me, because, you know, my mother is watching them, and if I don't come home by 10:00." Before Phil could respond, she began to walk out of the suddenly claustrophobic, snack room. Gloria felt no knee pain on the walk back to class. In fact, Phil could barely keep up with her.

Gloria had a hard time focusing on the material in class for the rest of the evening. The moment the professor released them, she tried to bolt for the door, but Phil was too fast. He intercepted her just as she reached the hallway, and before she could say anything, he said, "Look, I'm sorry I got a little confrontational, it certainly wasn't my intent."

Gloria smiled a polite smile and said, "It's OK, Phil, I wasn't offended, and a little debate is good for the mind."

He smiled back and added, "I'm glad you feel that way, and I just wanted to let you know that I'm still going to the Trolley Stop on the way home. If you feel like it, I would love to finish our discussion." He paused for a response, but when the only one he got was Gloria's deer-in-the-headlights expression, he continued, "If not, see you next class."

"See you next class, Phil."

Gloria arrived home at 9:50. When she opened the door, unusual quiet and the smell of herbal tea brewing on the stove greeted her. She laid her schoolbag down and sat at the kitchen table just as Hugh's mom entered from the dining room. In Gloria's eyes, Judy Glendenning was a saint. Since she had met Hugh, Judy was the antithesis of the stereotypical mother-in-law. She had been Gloria's anchor since Hugh's death, and by babysitting her two children, had simplified Gloria's return to school more than she knew. This was why Gloria had told Phil her mom was babysitting; because in her eyes, Judy was more of a mother than her own had ever been.

Judy sat at the table in the chair next to her and brushed a wisp of hair out of Gloria's eyes. "You look tired, Hon. Long day?"

All the way home, Gloria had deliberated over whether to tell her mother-in-law about Phil. Before she really made up her mind, she heard herself saying the words, "Long and strange, Mom. Would you believe a guy in my class asked me out tonight?"

Judy's eyes widened in a look of mock surprise and she said, "Why wouldn't I believe it, Gloria?"

"Well, you know, Hugh's barely gone two years, and it just feels weird that someone sees me that way."

Judy began to stare at Gloria intensely, and then she stood up from her chair and began to walk around Gloria as if inspecting her for something. "I'm sorry, Gloria, you must have left it in the car." Gloria looked at her, puzzled. Her mother-in-law continued, "You know, the sign announcing the date on which you lost your husband. I know you must wear one, how else would you expect other people to know."

Before Gloria could formulate a logical response, Judy walked to the stove, poured two cups of the herbal tea she had been brewing, and brought them to the table. She then sat down and gazed at Gloria. Gloria did not return her look; instead she stared into her tea and fidgeted with it. After some time, she met Judy's stare, but could only muster a mildly peevish, "What?"

Judy Glendenning leaned closer and said, "So, tell me about him."

Gloria felt her heart thumping in her chest. Not only was she considering "cheating" on Hugh, she was now about to discuss the details with his mother. She closed her eyes for a moment and reopened them, sure that she would wake up from this most surreal of nightmares. No such luck; Judy was still there, still wearing that pleasant, expectant smile. Reluctantly, Gloria began, "He's tall and a bit, umm, heavyset, but he's cute. Of course, not as cute as Hugh."

Judy smiled unctuously and added, "Of course he's not, how could anyone be?"

Rolling her eyes in feigned annoyance, Gloria continued, "He seems to have a good sense of humor, but he's a bit shy. I know it took a lot for him to approach me, and I am flattered by that." Her voice then rose a few octaves as she continued, "And after all, he's only asking to meet me at a local place where a lot of the people in our class congregate on Thursdays after class anyway, so it's pretty safe. And if it doesn't work out, it's not like I promised to marry him. Why am I making such a big deal out of this?"

Judy walked over and hugged her daughter-in-law and said, "Doesn't sound like you're sticking your neck out too far." Gloria felt relieved at this and a few tears meandered down her cheeks. It was not the decision to see another man that she felt conflicted about; it was the fact that by doing so, she was finally moving on and letting go. As if she was finally admitting to herself that Hugh was really gone forever.

Judy seemed to sense this and said, "You know, I remember the first night Hugh met you. He raved about this new girl he had met, and how she made him feel differently than any other girl he had ever known. He said he felt like his need to constantly see who was over the next horizon was gone. After he proposed to you, he used to laugh about the fact that he had gotten down on one knee, like in the movies. When I asked him why he did it, he said it just felt right, not corny at all. Then the night before you guys got married, he said the most remarkable thing; he said that he was not the most important person in his life any more. Now don't you think that same person would want you to be happy?"

Judy's words unlocked images from the depths of Gloria's memory, faded snapshots of that balmy afternoon when Hugh had proposed to her. These were memories she had dared not touch since his death. In an instant, she could feel the warm afternoon sun and the breeze caressing her. Sounds of birds chirping and leaves rustling in the gentle breeze came through loud and clear, and there, kneeling on one knee before her, was the man for whom she felt this impossible love, asking her to never leave him. With tears freely streaming down her face, Gloria said, "I'll tell you one thing,

Mom, if I do get married again, I'm not settling for any less than what I had."

As Gloria continued to sob, Judy retrieved a tissue from a dispenser on the counter, dabbed at Gloria's tear-streaked cheeks and said, "Crying's good sweetheart. Sometimes, you need to feel the anguish. In fact, you need to feel all the feelings, even the guilt. It's the only way you'll be able to let them go, and move on with your life. Remember, Gloria, you're still young, and picking up with your life is the most natural thing you can do."

A wan, almost resigned, smile crossed Gloria's face, and Judy continued, "Don't worry, no matter what happens, I will always be your kids' grandmother, and as such, I will meddle in your life as long as God gives me breath." Gloria looked up and saw the twinkle in her mother-in-law's eyes, and by degrees, her tears became interspersed with laughter.

The next class went slowly, and Phil did not approach Gloria during the break. She overheard him telling one of the other students that he would be going to his car for a CD with a beta version of some new computer game they had been discussing. She felt a little disappointed, but thought she would just talk to him after class. No such luck. When class ended, Phil was out the door and halfway to the stairs before she could even leave her seat.

Feeling a little dejected, she left class and walked to her car. As she drove out of the parking lot, she took a left turn, instead of the usual right, so as to pass the Trolley Stop. She didn't know why she did this, because she didn't know what kind of car Phil drove anyway. As she drew nearer to the bar, she was overtaken by a sudden whim. Almost involuntarily, she found herself turning into the parking lot, and, before she could talk herself out of it, she pushed through the front door and found herself standing in the foyer of the barroom, peering into the relative darkness of the interior.

The Trolley Stop was a small corner bar that had just been bought by a former business student of the college. He had remodeled it into a warm cheerful space with dark wood wainscoting topped by rough-hewn, off-white, plaster walls, a centrally located cherry wood bar and booths along all the walls. There was also plenty of paraphernalia adorning said walls, and hanging from the exposed rafters and stamped-metal ceiling. Gloria instantly felt at home here, and could see why it was so popular with a great majority of the students. As she wandered through, she saw a few people she vaguely knew from class. Finally, off in a corner booth by himself, she saw Phil. He had a bottle of beer in front of him and the textbook from their class open on the table. He seemed to be quite engrossed in it. Taking a deep breath, Gloria started toward the booth, and oddly, the Apollo 11, Neil Armstrong comment, "One small step for man, one giant leap for mankind," kept running through her mind as she approached him.

When she reached the table, Phil didn't bother to look up, instead he said, "Hi, thanks, I'll have another Millie's Evil Brew."

Gloria smirked and replied, "Hmm, that looks like about 150 calories, I could go for one myself if someone invited me to sit down." Phil looked up, a bit startled, but then the look gave way to a broad grin that told her she needn't have worried that he had changed his mind.

The conversation that ensued ranged from Gloria's widowed status and career change, to the whys and wherefores behind Phil's lack of dating experience and consequent chronic bachelorhood, his orphaned childhood, and finally, to the subject of weight-loss. Phil was still of the mind that calorie counting involved a huge life style change, and great tedium, and despite her most impassioned and detailed explanation, replete with examples, Gloria couldn't dissuade Phil of this notion. Of course, we all know Gloria could have talked until the bartender called "last call", and Phil would never have admitted to understanding the concepts of the diet. He was, after all, trying to create a reason for Gloria to give him another more intimate consultation, a date if you will. His intention became obvious when he finally suggested a field trip of sorts. He would take Gloria for an all-expense-paid dinner for two, during which she could demonstrate the ease of her approach to him. She caught the twinkle in his eye as he waited for her response, and she said, "Phil, that sounds a lot like you're asking me to go on a date with you."

"Well, if you promise not to run," Phil was referencing his first attempt at getting together with her, "then yes, I'm asking you for a date." Gloria smiled broadly and then playfully punched him on the arm just as a waitress arrived. After they ordered two more Millie's Evil Brews, Phil asked, "How did you know the calories in this particular beer?"

"I don't actually know the exact calorie count of this beer, but since it's not a light beer, it's probably in the one-hundred-fifty calorie per bottle range. If I'm off by ten or fifteen calories, it's not a big deal." She paused for a second to let her words sink in, and then said, "Get it?"

Suddenly, a look of epiphany crossed his face, and he said, "Maybe I've been making this too hard?" Gloria returned his rhetorical question with a nod and a smile, and thought, '*He gets it.*'

That Saturday, Phil and Gloria had their first date. Phil picked a local restaurant famous for their steaks. He was very curious to see if Gloria would blow her diet, and if not, what she would order from the restaurant's decidedly unlight menu.

For her first date with an unmarried man in over ten years, Gloria wore a cream-colored cotton sweater and khaki chinos that were subtle, but still flattered her new curves. Phil wore blue jeans with a light green shirt and what appeared to be a blueish green blazer. She laughed when she tried to compliment him on the color of his "blue-green" sport coat and she was admonished with a stern, "The color's sea-froth!" Gloria was beginning to really like his sense of humor. Phil's only sin was not opening and holding the door for Gloria when they entered the restaurant.

Even though Gloria did not believe in the diamond in the rough theory, she thought since, by his own admission, he had not dated much in his life, just this once, she would give him a little help by saying rather loudly, "UH, excuse me!"

Phil spun around at her query and managed a, "Whut?"

"Unless he has some war injury that prevents him from doing it, a gentleman always holds the door for a lady." At once, he turned red, and in a flurry of apology, he ran to get the door.

"Gloria, I'm so stupid, I mean I just didn't think, you know I'm really not good at this. I just know I could be. Please say I didn't blow it."

Still outside the door, she gave him a look of mock admonition and said, "We'll just have to see how the rest of the night goes." Phil looked at her with a wide-eyed-little-boy look that broke down her resolve and she couldn't help but smile. A look of relief passed over his features and then she said sternly, "Just don't let it happen again." Phil stood at attention as she passed through the door. Later, when Gloria related this incident to her mother-in-law, Judy Glendenning laughed until her eyes teared, even as she defended Phil, noting his orphaned upbringing.

The restaurant had an open airy feel to it. The waitress was very cheerful, and Gloria was surprised at how quickly she got over her case of nerves. For a before-dinner drink, she ordered a glass of wine, and Phil ordered an imported beer. At first, they talked mostly about class and their respective careers, but the conversation eventually shifted to how one could go to a restaurant and stay on any kind of diet, much less a calorically restricted one.

Phil asked, "So, not to bring up a sore subject, but how many calories are in that wine?"

"It's OK, Phil, I know that is the supposed reason for coming here. Wine is approximately 20 calories per ounce, so this glass is roughly 120 calories."

"How about my beer? Oh wait, roughly 150 calories, right?"

"Give or take maybe ten calories."

"Is that a lot for me?

"Given your size, Phil, I would say you probably need 2600 to 2700 calories per day to maintain your weight, so in that context..."

Suddenly, he interrupted her and said, "So, may I infer that I can drink a reasonable amount of beer and still lose weight?"

"The operative word is reasonable, but yes you may."

A look of what could only be called jubilance crossed his face, and he said, "All my diets before were all-or-nothing affairs, where I would swear something or many things off for the duration. This seems too easy."

She laughed and said, "I know what you mean. Swearing things off or vowing to starve myself for some arbitrary time period never worked for me either. I remember one low-fat diet I tried where I actually dreamed I was in prison and I was the only one not allowed to eat a cheeseburger." She chuckled again, "Believe me, when I went off that diet, I ate, uh, let's just say more cheeseburgers than I probably needed."

Phil's next surprise came after he ordered his dinner. Since he thought this might be the last time he could splurge, he ordered a nine-ounce steak, baked potato, and house salad with Russian dressing. He also ordered an appetizer consisting of sautéed shrimp over a bed of rice. Gloria ordered a seven-ounce steak with a baked potato and a salad with Russian dressing as well, but she ordered her dressing on the side. When she was done ordering, Phil shook his head and said, "I don't want to be a bad influence on you." She raised her eyebrows inquisitively. He continued, "I mean, I don't want you to go off your diet just because I'm splurging a little tonight."

She smiled and retorted, "Don't worry about me."

"No really, you've done such a good job, and I know you must have been so disciplined to get as far as you have, and I don't want to be the one who tempts you into blowing your diet."

'Someone's being a little presumptuous,' she thought, but then she realized she was being overly sensitive and she responded evenly, "Phil, I appreciate your concern, but really, I am not violating any of my rules."

"I hope I'm not breaching any boundaries or trusts here, but what is your calorie limit?"

"Well, for my size and activity, it works out to around 2000 calories per day."

Shaking his head, he said, "Oh, that doesn't sound too bad."

"That's what I've been trying to tell you."

"I think I will try this, uhh, starting tomorrow."

"Why not start it now?"

"I don't know how many calories I've eaten today."

"OK, what have you eaten today?"

Just two fast-food cheeseburgers, small fries, and a small coke."

"That's all?"

"Isn't that enough, he said?"

"Well, that totals to approximately 1000 calories, so based on what I said before, you've got around 1700 calories left for the day."

"OK, so I need 2700 calories to maintain weight, how do I use this approach to lose weight?

"Simple, never eat more than your 2700 calories, and on three or four days per week, eat some number of calories less than that."

"How much less?"

"It depends on how much you want to lose each week. For the sake of our little discussion, let's say, that's a pound per week. One easy way you could do it would be to just cut your intake to half of your daily caloric need on some number of days. So, in your case, it would be 2700 divided by two, which is 1350 calories per day. If you do this, you will be removing 1350 calories from your diet each day, so to lose what would actually amount to a little more than a pound, you would only need to this three days in a given week."

She could almost see the wheels turning in his head and he said, "What did I order just now, I mean with respect to calories?"

"Since you're splitting that shrimp appetizer with me, you're around 1200 with everything."

"So that means I can have dessert."

"Possibly, or another beer or two."

He smiled broadly again and said, "Ok, let's start now."

When they were ready to leave, Phil stood up and remarked how good he felt. He said, "This is the first time I can remember leaving a restaurant full, but not stuffed." He looked at her with a gleam in his eye and said, "Since I have calories left for two more beers, would you like to go dancing and burn off some dinner?"

A look of doubt crossed her face and she said, "Can computer people dance?"

He looked at her dourly and said, "Get ready to witness something not seen since the 1970s."

"Phil, walking works just as well as dancing to burn calories. I mean, we don't have to dance."

"Sorry, I'm committed!"

They left and went to a local nightclub that catered to people a little more chronologically challenged than one might find at a more typical establishment. The many meanings of the word "committed" resounded through Gloria's thoughts as she dutifully danced with Phil. Afterwards, when queried by co-workers, neither Phil nor Gloria would comment on his dancing, but perhaps Gloria's look of anguish when the subject was raised was all the comment needed. Oh well, they do have another date, so it mustn't have been that bad.

Phil's next fitness hurdle will be learning to exercise. Gloria knows this hurdle exists largely in his mind, and her next big job will be to make him see this too. Before we see how Gloria helps break down Phil's preconceptions, let's take a look at exactly how you would use a Part-Time caloric method, and how easy it can be.

As observed in the previous chapter, the subject of calorie counting can invoke long faces and comments like, "I can't be bothered to count calories, it's too much trouble," or "too tedious" or some similar response. Twenty-five years ago, we would have agreed. Today, however, with the advent of labeling most foods, it is easier than ever to keep track of one's caloric intake, so our first tip is to simply read the label if your food has one. Incidentally, McDonalds® has recently announced that its wrappers will soon have caloric values and other nutritional information printed on them. It will probably not be long before other eateries follow suit.

Of course, not everything is labeled, so you might want to go out and buy a book that lists the caloric values of foods, otherwise known as a calorie counter. These usually list other attributes of common foods like fat, protein, carbohydrate and vitamin and mineral content. Many of these also list the values of fast food. Yes, you can eat fast food as long as you observe the four rules enumerated back in chapter two. Fast food by itself does not make you fat. It does tend to be calorically dense, but, again, if your schedule has you eating at a fast food restaurant twice a week, the fact is, you can do it and still lose weight.

As an alternative or supplement to the calorie counter, there is always the Internet. If you happen to buy a book that does not list fast foods, you can usually get nutritional information from the company website, and it is often printable. Just go to the Internet and perform a search on the restaurant's name, and that will usually get you to their website. A little more surfing will usually take you to the page with the nutritional values. This actually has an advantage over a printed book in that it tends to be more up-to-date, so if a company has added new items to their menu, their nutritional values will be listed here in a more timely fashion.

If you are like most people, you will find that you tend to eat pretty much the same things on a week-to-week basis. This is good because within a few weeks, you will have ingrained into your memory banks the values for most things that you typically eat. An offshoot of this is that you can develop your own recipes for things that you commonly eat. As long as you make the item the same way every time, you will only have to add up the calories once. For instance, suppose you make a tuna sandwich with light bread, one tablespoon of light mayo, half of a six-ounce can of tuna, lettuce and onion. After a little label reading, you will find that this recipe works out to 228 calories. In actual practice, this would be rounded up to 250. If you know you've rounded things up a few times during a given day, you don't have to worry about counting every last creamer you put in your coffee. Just a little tip.

Is it starting to seem that the tedium of counting calories really only lasts a short time? With a little bit of effort, you should find that calorie counting becomes automatic, and sort of fades into the background, right where it belongs.

'*All right*,' you might be thinking, 'that stuff works great when I'm at home, but life is not always predictable. What if I find myself in a situation where I am unfamiliar with the foods I'm being served?' One neat little trick you can use, after you have started to become familiar with common caloric values of foods, is that you can compare an unknown item with a known item to get you in the ballpark. For example, suppose you are in a restaurant and they are serving really great nine-ounce cheeseburgers. You'd love to have one, but you don't have any idea how many calories are in it. Well, maybe you do. Let's see, you might know that there are 525 calories in a typical four-ounce fast food burger. If you double that, you will have 1050 calories. Since the nine-ounce burger roll is not twice as big as the four-ouncer, and the amount of cheese will usually be roughly 50 percent more than the smaller burger, you can safely estimate that the absolute most the big burger will be is somewhat less than 1050 calories. If you add up the ingredients, it is more likely in the 900-950 range. Even a woman on a 2100-calorie per day diet can afford this if she arranges her schedule for it, and if it is unplanned, she can eat half and bag the rest. It will make a delicious treat for the next day's lunch or dinner. By now, you should be starting to see that the little bit of effort it takes to learn to count calories pays off in the power to eat just about anything you want if you just use a little portion discipline.

There is yet another, more general, way to stay the course while dealing with the vagaries of modern life. As previously touched upon, foods tend to fall into general categories or families for caloric value. This makes it unnecessary to memorize every last food in a given family. Once you are familiar with these averages, you can make a pretty good guesstimate of almost any meal.

For example, if you go to a steak house and order a salad with thousand island dressing, seven-ounce filet mignon, and a baked potato with butter on the side, the calculation would go like this: most creamy salad dressings have 120 calories per serving, most red meats fall into the 70 calorie per ounce range, large baked potatoes are roughly 250 calories, butter is 35 calories per pat, and bread, which usually comes with this type of meal, is roughly 70 calories per slice. Knowing this, you can calculate, with enough accuracy for the purposes of this diet, the number of calories in this meal. Remember, this was basically what Phil ate, albeit with a little bigger steak and a bottle of beer, on his first date with Gloria.

In this case, the total calories would be roughly 990, using one pat of butter on the potato, one on the bread, and one tablespoon of salad dressing. If you add another pat of butter, you are basically in the thousand-calorie range. For a man whose DCN is 3000 per day, this is a nice meal that easily fits into this approach. What about a woman who cannot eat this many calories at a sitting? A simple way to handle this is to, again, cut everything in half and bag the rest. Filet mignon and half a baked potato also make a nice lunch for the following day. She could have, also, just structured her meals that day to allow a thousand calories for dinner, or how about, one-person orders an appetizer and one orders the entrée, and when they arrive, you just split them. Any of these ideas will work just fine, as long as the four basic rules from chapter two are observed.

Some rather high calorie examples were used in this little illustration, to make the point that with a caloric approach and a little creativity, you can eat anything in moderation, and the word "no" will assume a much less prominent role in your new lifestyle.

Could the above example be cleaned up to lower the calories? You bet! All you have to do is skip the bread and ask for the dressing on the side – remember to dip your salad, not much point in getting the dressing on the side if you just dump it on, versus the cook dumping it on – and you can cut approximately 120 calories from this meal. Or, if you put the bread back in and order roasted vegetables, instead of the baked potato, you can subtract 285 for the potato and one pat of butter, and add in approximately 100 calories for the vegetables for a net saving of 185 calories. Now go ahead and have that glass of wine, the price is roughly 130 calories per glass.

What if you don't know how much of any given food is in your meal? What if you order chicken or salmon and the number of ounces is not written on the menu? For this quandary, there is yet another simple answer. So simple, and commonsensical, in fact, that even a television psychologist might resist browbeating his latest victims with it. Yes, ladies and gentlemen, the answer to your quandary is to simply, ASK! Just ask the waitress or waiter if they can find out for you. If they seem reluctant, just tell them that you have a medical condition and point out how difficult it is to tip them when you are on the floor writhing in pain, or retching into one of their restroom sinks. Seriously, most good wait-staff will not consider this too much of an imposition.

OK, all that stuff is great if you are familiar with all these foods, but what if you're not a walking encyclopedia of calories? No problem, to make these types of calculations a little easier, I have compiled a short list and a long list of common foods and average caloric values to help you estimate your caloric intake. For each food item in the long list, I have, where possible, given you a high, low, and average caloric value. If the item you are eating is on the big side for that particular item, then use the high figure. If it is a small variant of that food item, then you can use the low or average caloric value. For many items, the caloric range where the greatest number of items appeared is cited; this is not necessarily the same as the average caloric value for that food. If you are not sure if the item would be considered large or small for that food type, then using the calorie range where most items appear may be your best bet when guesstimating calories for it. I would recommend that you take the time to scan this list and become familiar with these averages. You will find that when you start actually looking up specific foods, this will help you to start recognizing trends in a given type of food.

If you know in advance that you will be going to a party or some other atypical situation, do a little research and find out how many calories are in the foods they will be serving. Going into a situation like this with a preset idea of what and how much you will be eating can really stifle the urge to binge, and still allow you to enjoy yourself.

Oh, I know you probably think it is a royal pain to phone your party thrower and just blatantly ask what they will be having? Well, who says you have to be blatant? After all, this might sound a little rude or ungrateful, as though your attendance might be contingent upon their proposed menu. Instead of straining your friendship that way, you could concoct a clever verbal dodge, as another fictitious friend of ours does here and say something like, "Hi Patina, this is Globella." (not their real names) "Listen Hon, I was just watching the stock market channel and they said that pork belly futures are trending up, and this could affect the prices at the supermarket as early as this weekend, so if you are planning on serving pork chops, pork loin, or bacon wrapped hotdogs at the party, you might want to buy them now to avoid the price spike that seems destined to ripple through the global pork market."

Notice the subtle beauty of this interrogatory. Instead of thinking, *'Hey, she just wants to know what we'll be serving,'* Patina was impressed by Globella's concern for her financial well-being, and cheerfully answered, "Why thank you, Globella, for being so thoughtful, but you needn't be concerned, as we will be serving hamburgers, hotdogs sans bacon, chicken wings, raw veggies with vegetable dip and fried mozzarella sticks." When Globella hangs up, not only has she gotten the answer to her query, but she has also added another low-cal dollop of glue to her friendship with Patina.

For those of you who might want a more conventional approach, you could simply call your host and offer to bring a dish. From there, it would be a short conversational segue to what might be on the menu, as well as to what other people are bringing. Some other advantages to this approach are that, since you will have control over what you are making, you will be sure to like at least one food at the party, and you will know how many calories are in it.

Hey, here's another little tip. If food is served in a sit-down manner, consent to only small portions and take at least 20 minutes to finish. If after 20 minutes, you are still hungry then seconds are probably OK, but this time, try to take only half as much as the first time.

What if it's served buffet style? All I can say is, if your hosts prefer to play fast and loose with their guests clothing budget and molecular structure, then you need to devote your full attention to the next two paragraphs. Yes, I said molecular structure. Just keep reading.

Buffet lines are pretty much anathema to most weight loss plans, and for good reason. C'mon, think about it, we've all known someone, maybe it even happened to you, who has literally doubled their weight in one visit to a buffet-style restaurant. The cost in new clothes alone can be devastating. Even worse, during my research for this book, I came across a very credible supermarket tabloid that reported one man who ate so much at a buffet style restaurant, that he collapsed in on himself, black hole style, and actually fell out of this universe, only to pop up in an alternate universe where spinach is eaten for dessert. Fact or fiction? You decide. Just to be safe though, I feel it is my duty to give you a workable strategy that will help keep your atoms "unsmashed" and obviate the necessity for before and after dinner clothes.

The first part of the strategy is to use your initial trip to the feed line to fill a plate with stuff you know is low-cal, like vegetables and a plain piece of protein such as baked or broiled fish or chicken. Second, as mentioned above, take at least 20 minutes to finish your first helping. This will give your blood sugar time to rise, and take the edge off of your appetite. Now, when you go back for the goodies, you will be much less likely to overdo it. This will also give your stomach time to expand and give you a nice full feeling on less calories, which brings us to the third and final prong in this attack: respect the full feeling. It's OK if you leave the restaurant while there is still food in the warming trays. Seriously, after you have used "The Part-Time Approach" for a while, your stomach will tend to shrink and make the full feeling a better gauge.

Although The Part-Time Diet Approach does not recommend any specific foods to eat or not eat, I would be remiss if I did not mention that this approach will work better if you moderate carbohydrates that have a high glycemic index. Glycemic index refers to how quickly a food is converted to blood sugar after you have eaten it, or how fast and how much it raises your blood sugar. The faster a food raises your blood sugar, the higher its glycemic index, for example, table sugar has a very high glycemic index. When you eat these foods, your body produces a lot of insulin very quickly. Insulin is a hormone that is great at storing any excess calories as body fat. It also quickly lowers blood sugar, which can goad one into eating excessively. To minimize this response, choose high fiber carbohydrates like: vegetables, nuts, whole grain breads and cereals, and limit highly refined carbohydrate foods like: white bread, candy, pasta made from white flour, bagels etc. Before anybody gets the idea that you can gorge on high-fiber carbohydrates with no regard for calorie content, let us squelch that idea right here. The body is very adept at storing any unused calories as fat, regardless of the source.

Now, you might be thinking that these are rules you can live with, but eventually everyone makes a mistake. What then? Do you hang your head in shame, and bleat out your pent up feelings of self-loathing to a talk radio psychologist, or does the "Part-Time Diet Approach" have a pragmatic way of handling the occasional tumble from the weight-loss wagon? You'll just have to keep reading to find out. OK, now let's see the lists.

A WORD ABOUT THESE LISTS

Remember, these lists are not meant to be exact or comprehensive. These averages are just meant to get you in the ballpark if you're in a situation where you may not have access to a calorie counter, or may be unfamiliar with a particular restaurant's cuisine. They are not exact for any given food item, and it is much simpler and more accurate to read labels or a calorie counter whenever possible.

NOW, AS PROMISED, THE LISTS, UHH AFTER THESE HANDY CONVERSIONS

> - 1 tablespoon is ½ ounce
> - 4 tablespoons is ¼ cup
> - 8 tablespoons is ½ cup
> - 3 teaspoons per tablespoon
> - 100 grams is equal to 3.5 ounces
> - Women, a meat, chicken or fish patty about the size of your fist is three and a half to four ounces. Men, it's closer to five ounces.

FINALLY, A QUICK LIST OF DOWN AND DIRTY AVERAGES FOR COMMON FOODS

Beans and Legumes – You know, like chickpeas in a salad, these usually run in the 36-calorie per ounce range, watch out for Navy beans, they can run 100 calories per ounce.

Cheese – Mostly runs in the 100-calorie per ounce range, or 66 calories per slice.

Bread – Usually runs in the 60 - 75-calorie per slice range, light bread runs around 40 calories per slice.

Cream Sauces – *When not running down the front of my shirt*, these usually run around 120 calories per tablespoon.

Eggs – Large chicken eggs are 80 calories, 60 calories for the yolk and 20 for the white. Hint: Want to make a great low calorie breakfast? Take three eggs, throw away two yolks and add two ounces of skim milk and an ounce of American cheese. Use a pat of butter to grease the pan. The three eggs minus two yolks add up to 120 calories. The cheese is 100 calories, and the butter is 35. Don't forget to add 20 calories for the skim milk. Totaling it up, we see that for 275 calories, you have a great tasting omelet. Add a slice of low-cal bread with another pat of butter and you come up with another 75 calories. How about some orange juice? Six ounces will cost you another 100 calories. Grand total for this breakfast is 450 calories. Not a bad way to start even a 1200-calorie day.

Fish – Usually runs in the 50-calorie per ounce range; fry it and you double the calories.

Lentils –Run around 100 calories per ounce.

Nuts –Run in the 180 calories per ounce range.

Peas – Run around 100 calories per ounce.

Potato Chips and Snacks Fried in Oil – Average 150 calories per ounce.

Poultry – Usually runs in the 60-calorie per ounce range, if you fry it you basically double the calories, and breading adds even more.

Pretzels and Baked Snacks – Usually run in the 110 – 120-calorie per ounce range.

Red Meat – Basically, 70 calories per ounce, although leaner cuts are less, this is still a good rule of thumb.

Salad Dressing – Oily dressing is roughly 100 calories per tablespoon, light varieties often run half of this, or 50 calories per tablespoon.

Soda – Regular usually runs in the 150-calorie per 12-ounce can range.

Vegetables, Non-Starchy – Although they do have calories, the amount is low enough that you really don't even need to count them, but beware the butter.

Vegetables, Starchy – An example would be potatoes, which are approximately 20 calories per ounce.

LONG LIST OF DOWN AND DIRTY AVERAGES OF COMMON FOODS

All caloric values used in these averages are from the nutrition.gov website's great and free downloadable database, or from the manufacturer's labels. They are not meant to be exact, they are just meant to give you a sense of the caloric content of typical foods.

| BEVERAGES, ALCOHOLIC

(distilled) including gin, rum, vodka and whiskey

❖ *80 proof* – has 64 calories per ounce, or 96 per jigger
       (a jigger is 1.5 ounces)
❖ *86 proof* – has 69 calories per ounce, or 104 per jigger
❖ *90 proof* – has 73 calories per ounce, or 110 per jigger
❖ *94 proof* – has 76 calories per ounce, or 114 per jigger
❖ *100 proof* – has 82 calories per ounce, or 123 per jigger

Beer
Most frequently contains 150 calories per 12-ounce serving, with a few imported brands going as high as 190 calories.

Light Beer
Ranges from 95 to 120 calories per 12-ounce serving, these are usually labeled.

Selected Mixed Drinks
Mixed drinks are mostly some combination of distilled alcohol and a mixer, or flavoring. The mixers tend to be high in sugar, so go light on these drinks. Caloric values quoted here are for a typical serving size that you could expect to be served in a public bar or restaurant. This is usually a four-ounce drink with one jigger of alcohol per serving. .

- ❖ *Bloody Mary* – 124 calories per serving
- ❖ *Bourbon and Soda* – 160 calories per serving, calories can be reduced significantly by using diet soda
- ❖ *Daiquiri* – 225 calories per serving, although some recipes double this figure
- ❖ *Margarita* – 234 calories per 3.4 ounce serving
- ❖ *Martini* – 274 calories per serving
- ❖ *Pina Colada* – 219 calories per serving
- ❖ *Rum & Coke* – 150 calories per serving
- ❖ *Scotch & Soda* - 150 calories per serving
- ❖ *Seven and Seven* – 150 calories per serving
- ❖ *Sloe Gin Fizz* – 140 calories per serving
- ❖ *Vodka Gimlet* – 110 calories per serving
- ❖ *Vodka or Gin & Tonic* – 140 calories per serving
- ❖ *Whiskey Sour* (No garnish) – 193 calories per serving
- ❖ *White Russian* – 240 calories per serving.

Basically, drinks with cream and/or sugar average around 250 calories per serving, while those without average 145.

Wine
Averages roughly 130 calories per six-ounce glass, light wine is around 90 calories per six-ounce glass.

Wine Cooler
These typically run an average of 215 calories per serving.

SOFTER, FRIENDLIER, MORE COMPASSIONATE BEVERAGES

Cocoa Mixes
These average 93 calories per serving among 31 items surveyed, with a high of 150 and a low of 25 calories. Fortunately, most of these are labeled.

Coffee Drinks
Regular coffee has essentially no calories by itself. The following caloric values are for the creams, etc. that can be used to flavor coffee like cappuccino, vanilla or amaretto, and that sort of thing. Average is 77 calories per serving, which as near as we can tell is two tablespoons. Among 29 items surveyed, the high was 170 and a low was 30 calories. Sadly, those little flavored coffee creamers in your local convenience store are roughly 40 calories per item. *Ouch!*

Fruit Juice, Vegetable Juice and Juice Drinks
Apple juice and orange juice run 120 calories per eight-ounce serving. Grape juice runs 160 calories per eight-ounce serving. The average for fruit juice is roughly 130 calories per eight-ounce serving among 305 items surveyed, with a low of 30 calories for one of the light variants, and a high of 180 calories. Fruit juices with high sugar content tend to run higher. Vegetable juices tend to run toward the bottom of the range, with an average of 57 calories per eight-ounce serving.

Mixers
These are things like Bloody Mary and Pina Colada mix, and average 102 calories among 23 items, with a range from 10 to 180 calories for an eight-ounce serving. The greatest number of items fall between 80 and 100 calories.

Nutritional Drinks
These include things like Slim Fast, Weight Watchers and other meal replacement drinks. The serving size is eight ounces. The average is 168 calories among 450 items, ranging between 80 and 360 calories, with the greatest number of items falling between 190 and 220 calories.

Carbonated Soft Drinks

These are sugar-sweetened drinks including soda and some soda mixed with fruit juice drinks. The average for an eight-ounce serving is 113 calories over 91 items, with a range between 90 and 220 calories, and the greatest number of items falling between 110 and 130 calories. A typical 12-ounce can of sugar-sweetened soda is 150 calories. The diet variants average less than five calories per serving.

Non-Carbonated Soft Drinks

These are drinks like Kool Aid®. They average 100 calories per eight-ounce serving over 58 items, with a range between 60 and 230 calories. The greatest number of items falls between 110 to 130 calories. Read the labels!

Sports Drinks

These drinks average 79 calories per eight-ounce drink with a range between 50 and 193 calories. The greatest number of items falls between 60 and 70 calories. There is only one item falling into the 193-calorie category, so the average here is pretty typical of what one might see.

Tea Drinks

These drinks average 94 calories per eight-ounce serving over 22 items, with a range between 60 and 140 calories, and the greatest number of items falling into the 80 to 90-calorie range.

Mineral Water

Sugar-sweetened varieties have an average of 205 calories per 12-ounce serving over seven items, with a range between 200 and 220 calories. Plain mineral water has no calories.

| BREADS AND OTHER BAKED STUFF

Bagel

The grocery store item is usually 175 calories. Bagels bought at specialty vendors can be in the 350-calorie range.

Biscuits
These average 92 calories per serving over six items, with a range between 59 and 127 calories. Most items appeared in the 90 - 120-calorie range. A serving is usually one biscuit.

Bread
Averages 70 calories per slice. This is the size of a regular slice of bread from a typical supermarket loaf, approximately one-half of an inch thick. Low calorie breads usually run in the 40 – 50-calorie per slice range.

Breadsticks
Small range in the 15-calorie per stick zone, and large are in the 45 – 90-calorie range, be careful, one brand is as high as 130 calories for one stick.

Breakfast or Sweet Rolls
These range from 60 to 500 calories, with an average of 244 calories over 58 items. Be careful with these, typically, store-bought items run to the high side of this average.

Cake
A serving is two ounces, or roughly a two-by-three-inch slice, unless otherwise stated.
- ❖ *Angelfood* – Averages 149 calories per serving.
- ❖ *Boston Cream Pie* – Averages 144 calories per serving.
- ❖ *Carrot*– Averages 237 calories per serving.
- ❖ *Cheese* - Averages 183 calories per serving.
- ❖ *Cherry Fudge* – Averages 150 calories per serving.
- ❖ *Chocolate* – Averages 221 calories per serving.
- ❖ *Coffee* - Averages 200 calories per serving.
- ❖ *Cupcakes* – Averages 160 calories per serving. A typical serving is one cup cake. These vary widely, for instance, Tasty Cake Cupcakes® are near the low end of the spectrum, which is 131 calories per cupcake.
- ❖ *Fruit* – Averages 185 calories per serving.
- ❖ *Gingerbread* – Averages 226 calories per serving.
- ❖ *Marble*– Averages 237 calories per serving.
- ❖ *Pineapple* – Averages 182 calories per serving.
- ❖ *Pound*– Averages 221 calories per serving. Fat-free runs roughly 161 calories per serving.

- ❖ *Short Cake* – Averages 197 calories per serving. *Does this imply the existence of a long cake?*
- ❖ *Sponge*– Averages 168 calories per serving.
- ❖ *Store Bought Snack Cakes* – These are basically big cupcakes, and Range from 130 to 360 calories with the average around 200 calories. Most of these are labeled.
- ❖ *White/Yellow* – Averages 227 calories per serving.

Cookies
Average 79 calories per serving over 320 items, with a range between 6 and 360 calories. Most items appeared in the 50–60-calorie range. A serving is an average-sized cookie. Think the size of an Oreo®. Bigger cookies, sadly, fall into the higher end of the range. If an Oreo® falls into the 60-calorie range, then a cookie that's twice as big probably contains twice the calories. Cookies with nuts also tend to run to the high end of the range.

Crackers
Average 10 calories per serving over 109 items, with a range between 2 and 19 calories. A serving is one small cracker, approximately one-by-one inch. Bigger crackers fall into a higher range, averaging 41 calories per serving over 42 items, with a range between 11 and 120. Most items fall into the 25 – 50 range.

Cracker Sandwiches
Average 181 calories per serving over 19 items, with a range between 130 and 230 calories. Most items appeared in the 190-calorie range. A serving is usually 1 package.

Crumpets
Allow us to trumpet, if you love a good crumpet, no need to dump it, since cals are just a hundrit. That's 100 calories for the poetically challenged.

Doughnuts
Average 190 calories per serving over five items, with a range between 162 and 219 calories. Most items appeared in the 200-calorie range. A serving is one three-inch diameter doughnut. Doughnuts ranging in the 3 3/4-inch diameter run in the 250-calorie range. Bigger doughnuts equal more calories. Specialty retailers usually run around 350 calories per item. Good

news! Krispy Kreme® only run around 200 for the plain glazed doughnuts. Doughnuts with filling run into the 300-plus range.

English Muffins
Average approximately 160 calories per muffin, to as high as 250 calories for the stuffed or fancier muffins. Remember, check labels, despite what is in this database, we have seen these in the supermarket for as low as 120 calories per muffin.

Hamburger and Hotdog Rolls
Average in the 120-calorie range, again, if possible, read labels because some of the heavier rolls can go into the 230 range.

Muffins
These average 149 calories per muffin, with a range from 120 to 190 calories.

Pies
Average 365 calories per serving, with a range from 270 to 500 calories per serving, which is usually 1/8 of a nine-inch pie, or 1/6 of an eight-inch pie. *You might think these are more suitable for throwing than eating if you are trying to stay within a caloric budget, but like all other foods, if you really want it, you can have it OCCASIONALLY.*

Stuffing Mix
If you're eating Thanksgiving Dinner away from home, this could save you. These range from 60 to 170 calories per one-half cup, with an average of 117 calories for 34 different brands.

Shells for Tacos etc.
These range from 50 to 85 calories, with an average of 62 calories per item.

| BARS, CANDY ETC

Candy
Small bite-sized candies range around 25 calories per item. Watch out for the mid-sized candies with nuts, as they can range over 100 calories per item. The lesson learned here is that if you're at a party and find yourself

picking at these, be aware that they add up fast. Fortunately, most of these candies are labeled with regard to calories, and what constitutes a serving.

Candy Bars
Candy bars average 229 calories per regular-sized bar averaged over 33 items, with a range between 90 and 280 calories. The greatest number of items, however, falls into the 240-calorie range. Fortunately, today these are pretty much all labeled.

| CEREAL AND BREAKFAST STUFF

Breakfast Drinks
Average 157 calories per serving over 14 items, with a range between 70 and 220 calories. Most items appeared in the 200-calorie range. Servings vary; they are usually considered 10 ounces. Most are labeled.

Hot Cereal
Averages 142 calories per serving over 69 items, with a range between 100 and 220 calories. Most items appeared in the 150-calorie range. Servings vary; they are usually considered 1/4 to 1/3 cup or one packet. Most are labeled.

Cold Cereal
Averages 154 calories per serving over 289 items, with a range between 30 and 290 calories. Most items appeared in the 120-calorie range. Servings vary, but they are usually considered one-half cup to one cup. Most are labeled.

| DAIRY ITEMS

Butter
- ❖ *Regular* – Averages 100 calories per tablespoon.
- ❖ *Light* – Averages 50 calories per tablespoon.
- ❖ *Whipped* – Averages 60 calories per tablespoon. Whipping adds air to the butter, making it less dense, thus decreasing the caloric content versus regular.

❖ *Whipped Light* – Averages 35 calories per tablespoon.

Margarine

❖ *Regular* – Ranges between 80 – 100 calories per tablespoon.

❖ *Light* – Tends to range between 50 – 80 calories per tablespoon, with the vast majority of items in the 50 – 60-calorie range.

❖ *Low Fat* – Tends to range between 0 – 40 calories per tablespoon, with the vast majority of items in the 25-calorie range.

Cheese

❖ *Regular* – Averages 104 calories per serving over 108 items, with a range between 80 and 120 calories. Most items appeared in the 100–110-calorie range. A serving is usually one ounce. A typical slice of cheese is two-thirds of an ounce, so approximately 66 calories per slice.

❖ *Light* – Averages 66 calories per serving over 38 items, with a range between 45 and 80 calories. Most items appeared in the 60–70 calorie range. A serving is usually one ounce. A typical slice of cheese is two-thirds of an ounce, so approximately 45 calories per slice.

❖ *Cheese Product* – These run in the 80 – 90-calorie per ounce range.

❖ *Cheese Snacks and Spreads* – These most commonly fall into the 90 calories per two-tablespoon serving range.

❖ *Cottage Cheese* – Regular runs in the 110 – 120-calorie per one-half-cup range. Light, or 2% runs in the 90-calorie per one-half-cup range, and fat free runs in the 70-calorie per one half-cup range.

❖ *Cream Cheese* – Averages 92 calories per serving over 20 items, with a range between 60 and 110 calories. Most items appeared in the 90 – 100-alorie range. A serving is usually two tablespoons.

❖ *Light Cream Cheese* – Average 48 calories per two tablespoon serving over nine items, with a range between 25 and 70 calories. Most items appeared in the 25 – 50-calorie range.

❖ *Feta Cheese* – Averages 90 calories per one-ounce serving.

❖ *Goat Cheese* – Averages 80 calories per one-ounce serving over four items, with a range between 70 and 130 calories. Most items appeared in the 90 – 100-calorie range.

❖ *Mozzarella Cheese* – Averages roughly 80 calories per serving over seven items, with a range between 70 and 80 calories. This is the case because most of the items were 80 calories. A serving is usually one ounce.

❖ *Light Mozzarella Cheese* – Averages 52 calories per serving over seven items, with a range between 35 and 70 calories. Most items appeared in the 25 – 50-calorie range. A serving is usually one ounce.

❖ *Parmesan* – Averages 20 – 25 calories per one-ounce serving.

❖ *Ricotta* – Averages 100 – 110 calories per one-quarter cup.

❖ *Light Ricotta* – Averages 60 – 90 calories per one-quarter-cup serving.

❖ *Velveeta* – Averages 80 calories per ounce.

Cream
Averages 43 calories per serving over six items, with a range between 40 and 50 calories. A serving is usually one tablespoon.

Light Cream and Half & Half
Averages 20 calories per serving over six items, with a range between 10 and 30 calories. A serving is usually one tablespoon, or one-half ounce.

Eggnog
You probably don't want to know this, and you should have the kids leave the room because it is obscene, but here goes: Averages roughly 170 calories per **four-ounce** serving, **OMIGAWD!!**

Egg and Egg Substitutes
A large chicken egg is 80 calories with 60 coming from the yolk, and 20 from the egg white, egg *substitutes* run around 35 calories per one-quarter cup.

Milk
The following values are for cow's milk:
• *Whole Milk* - 150 calories per eight-fluid-ounce cup
• *Two% Milk* - 120 calories per eight-fluid-ounce cup
• *One% Milk* - 100 calories per eight-fluid-ounce cup
• *Skim Milk* - 80 calories per eight-fluid-ounce cup
• *Evaporated Milk* - 25 calories per two tablespoons
　　　　　　　　(approx. one ounce)

Sour Cream

Averages 60 calories per tablespoon, light varieties run around 35 calories.

Tofu

Averages 70 calories per three and one-half ounce serving.

Whipped Toppings

Averages 20 calories per serving over five items, with a range between 15 and 30 calories. A serving is usually two tablespoons.

Yogurt

In Philadelphia, this might be the way one would hail a woman named Gertrude, but for the rest of the country, this refers to a creamy foodstuff that averages 142 calories per serving over 175 items, with a range between 65 and 273 calories. Most items appeared in the 160–190-calorie range. A serving is usually six ounces. Non-fat items are lowest and hover in the 100 calories per serving range.

| FRUITS, CANNED OR BOTTLED

Of course, most bottled and canned foods will be labeled. They are mentioned here just to give you a general feel for how many calories are in a given food group. This instinct will come in handy if you are in a situation where you can't read a can or bottle, like in a restaurant or at a friend's house. Remember, restaurants tend to give larger servings to make the patron feel they have gotten their money's worth.

Apple Sauce

Averages 83 calories per serving, which is generally one-half cup, over 16 items, with a range between 50 and 110 calories. The greatest number of items falls into the 85-calorie range.

Canned Fruit

Averages 90 calories per one-half cup over 67 items, with a range between 45 and 250 calories, and the greatest number of items falling into the 80-calorie range. Since almost as many items fall into the 90-100-calorie range, the best estimate will usually be in the 90-calorie range. Pineapples tend to run between 60 and 90 calories for two slices. Calories are higher for slices in syrup.

FRUITS, RAW

- ❖ *Apple With Skin* – 80 calories / fruit
- ❖ *Apricot* – 20 calories / fruit
- ❖ *Avocado* – 150 calories / fruit
- ❖ *Banana* – 100 calories/fruit
- ❖ *Blackberry* – 60 calories / three-quarters cup
- ❖ *Cherry* – 50 calories / cup
- ❖ *Coconut* – 100 calories / ounce
- ❖ *Cranberry* – 25 calories / one-half cup
- ❖ *Elderberry* – 50 calories / one-half cup *(How do you get elderberries without youngerberries?)*
- ❖ *Fig* – 110 calories / cup *(Go FIGure)*
- ❖ *Grape* – 30 calories / 20 fruits
- ❖ *Grapefruit* – 50 calories / one-half fruit
- ❖ *Guava* – 45 calories / fruit
- ❖ *Kumquat* 15 calories / one-half cup
- ❖ *Lemon* – 20 calories / medium fruit
- ❖ *Lime* – 20 calories / fruit
- ❖ *Mango* – 130 calories / fruit
- ❖ *Melon, cantaloupe* – 60 calories / cup
- ❖ *Melon, casaba* – 45 calories / cup
- ❖ *Melon, honeydew* – 60 calories / cup
- ❖ *Nectarine* – 70 calories / fruit
- ❖ *Orange*, medium – 60 calories / fruit
- ❖ *Papaya* – 120 calories / fruit
- ❖ *Peach* – 40 calories / fruit
- ❖ *Pear* – 100 calories / fruit
- ❖ *Pineapple* – 80 calories / cup
- ❖ *Plantain* – 220 calories / fruit
- ❖ *Plum* – 35 calories / fruit
- ❖ *Pomegranate* – 100 calories / fruit
- ❖ *Raspberry* – 30 calories / one-half cup
- ❖ *Rhubarb* – 10 calories / one-half cup
- ❖ *Strawberry* – 45 calories / cup

❖ *Tangerine* – 40 calories / fruit
❖ *Watermelon* –50 calories / cup

| GRAINS

Pasta – Averages 37 calories per ounce after cooking.

Rice – White, cooked is approximately 37 calories per ounce or 200 per cup.

Rice – Brown, cooked is approximately 32 calories per ounce or 218 per cup.

These figures may seem a little out of kilter until you realize that cups measure volume and ounces measure weight. If you measure an ounce of white rice and an ounce of brown rice, you will see that the white rice takes up more space and therefore less fits in a cup, hence fewer calories in a cup.

| GRAVY AND GRAVY MIX

Remember, these are just the flavoring of these gravies, if butter or flour is added, these caloric values will go up accordingly with the added ingredients. Again, always read the manufacturer's label when possible.

❖ *Au Jus* – *Gesundheit!* Averages ten calories per one-quarter cup.
❖ *Beef and Brown Gravy* - Averages 16 calories per serving over 13 items, with a range between 5 and 30 calories. Most items appeared in the 25-calorie range. A serving is usually one-quarter cup.
❖ *Chicken Gravy* – Averages 25 calories per serving over 13 items, with a range between 10 and 45 calories. Most items appeared in the 25-calorie range. A serving is usually one-quarter cup.
❖ *Home-Style Gravy Mix* – Averages 12 calories per serving over five items, with a range between 10 and 15 calories. Servings vary; most commonly they are usually considered one-quarter package.
❖ *Mushroom Gravy* – Averages 23 calories per serving over seven items, with a range between 10 and 60 calories. Most items

appeared in the 25-calorie range. Servings vary. Most commonly they are considered one-quarter cup.

❖ *Onion Gravy Mix* – Averages roughly 22 calories per serving over five items, with a range between 10 and 25 calories. A serving is usually one-quarter cup or two ounces.

❖ *Pork Gravy* – Averages roughly 22 calories per serving over three items, with a range between 10 and 45 calories. A serving is usually one-quarter cup or two ounces.

❖ *Sausage, Stroganoff, Steak, and Turkey Gravy* - Averages 25 calories per serving over seven items, with a range between 15 and 35 calories. Most items appeared in the 25-calorie range. Servings vary; they are usually considered one-quarter cup, or one-quarter package.

MEAT AND POULTRY

Unless otherwise mentioned, the serving size will be three ounces after cooking.

Ground Meats:
❖ *95 percent lean* – approximately 50 calories per ounce.
❖ *90 percent lean* – approximately 60 calories per ounce.
❖ *85 percent lean* – approximately 70 calories per ounce.
❖ *80 percent lean* – approximately 75 calories per ounce.
❖ *75 percent lean* – approximately 80 calories per ounce.

Organ Meats:
❖ *Brain* – 50 calories per ounce *Probably one of the smartest things you can eat.*
❖ *Heart* – 44 calories per ounce.
❖ *Kidney* – 43 calories per ounce.
❖ *Liver* – 50 calories per ounce.

Ribs
Averages 264 calories per serving, or 88 calories per ounce, over 43 items, with a range between 170 and 400 calories. Most items appeared in the 300 - 350-calorie range for a serving of three ounces of meat (think the size of an

average female fist). Marbled run to the higher end of the range, or stated another way, leaner ribs mean less calories.

Round
Averages 175 calories per serving, or 60 calories per ounce, with fat trimmed, over 39 items, with a range between 130 and 250 calories. Most items appeared in the 160 - 190-calorie range. A serving is usually three ounces (think the size of an average female fist). Leaner cuts have fewer calories.

Short Loin, Tenderloin
Otherwise known as filet mignon, averages 224 calories per serving, or 74 calories per ounce, with fat trimmed, over 12 items, with a range between 170-300 calories per serving. A serving is usually three ounces (think as big as the average female fist). Leaner cuts have fewer calories, so trim the fat.

Short Loin, Top Loin, and Top Sirloin
Averages 202 calories per serving, or 67 calories per ounce, with fat trimmed, over 17 items with a range between 160 and 300 calories per serving. Most items appeared in the 160 – 190-calorie range. A serving is usually three ounces (think as big as the average female fist). Leaner cuts have fewer calories.

Chicken, Meat Only
Averages 156 calories per three-ounce serving, (think as big as the average female fist) or 52 calories per ounce, over 23 items, with a range between 130 and 200 calories. Most items appeared in the 130 – 160-calorie per serving range. White meat runs a few calories less than dark meat.

Chicken Meat and Skin
Averages 202 calories per three-ounce serving. Think as big as the average female fist, or 67 calories per ounce, over 25 items, with a range between 160 and 260 calories. Most items appeared in the 190 – 220-calorie per serving range. White meat runs a few calories less than dark meat.

Ham
Averages 140 calories per three-ounce serving, or 46 calories per ounce, over 23 items, with a range between 80 and 230 calories. Most items

appeared in the 160 – 190-calorie per serving range. Lean ham or ham with little marbling runs toward the lower end of the range.

Pork Loin
Averages 199 calories per 3.5-ounce serving, or 56 calories per ounce, over 63 items, with a range between 140 and 290 calories per serving. Most items appeared in the 160 – 190-calorie per serving range. Leaner is lower. Many products are labeled.

Pork Shoulder
Averages 220 calories per 3.5-ounce serving, or 62 calories per ounce, over 15 items, with a range between 140 and 280 calories. Most items appeared in the 190 – 250-calorie per serving range. Leaner is lower.

Turkey White Meat
Averages 90 calories per three-ounce serving, or 30 calories per ounce, over 21 items, with a range between 72 and 130 calories. Most items appeared in the 71 – 80-calorie per serving range. Leaner is lower.

Turkey Dark Meat
Averages 140 calories per three-ounce serving, or 46 calories per ounce, over six items, with a range between 110 and 170 calories. Most items appeared in the 130-170-calorie per serving range. Leaner is lower.

Veal
Averages 170 calories per three-ounce serving, or 56 calories per ounce, over 32 items, with a range between 130 and 240 calories. Most items appeared in the 160 – 190-calorie per serving range. Leaner is lower.

| MEATS, PACKAGED AND LUNCHEON

Canned Meat and Poultry
Average is 110 calories per serving over 26 items, with a range between 50 and 390 calories, and the greatest number of items falling into the 100-calorie range. A serving here is roughly two to three ounces. Practically all of these are labeled these days.

Bacon
Averages 36 calories per serving over 18 items, with a range between 23 and 50 calories. Most items appeared in the 25 – 50-calorie range. A serving is usually one slice.

Breakfast Sausage
Averages 79 calories per serving over 35 items, with a range between 39 and 150 calories. Most items appeared in the 60 – 90-calorie range. A serving is usually one link or patty. Pork runs to the high side of the range, turkey runs to the low side. *True story: I once knew a family with a son named Lincoln and a daughter named Patricia, and yes, they called them Linc and Patty. Parents, please refrain from branding your children with permanent monikers if your blood alcohol level exceeds the legal limit for operating a motor vehicle in your state, or your capacity for foresight has been otherwise impaired!! This message has been brought to you by B.A.F.O.O.N. (Ban All Funny Odd Offspring Names.)*

Frankfurters
Average 123 calories per serving over 25 items, with a range between 39 and 185 calories. Most items appeared in the 130 – 160-calorie range. A serving is usually one hot dog. Pork runs to the high side of the range, turkey runs to the low side. A typical beef hot dog with bun runs from 250 – 300 calories.

Luncheon Meats
Many of these tend to run higher than the 70-calorie per ounce typical for red meat, because of their high fat content.

- ❖ *Bologna, Beef and Pork* – Averages 89 calories per serving over six items, with a range between 86 and 94 calories. A serving is usually one ounce, or a medium thickness slice.
- ❖ *Bologna, Light Beef and Pork* – Averages 61 calories per serving over five items, with a range between 56 and 64 calories. A serving is usually one ounce, or a medium thickness slice.
- ❖ *Bologna, Chicken and Turkey* – These can run in the 50 – 75 calories per serving range. A serving is usually one ounce, or a medium thickness slice.
- ❖ *Braunschweiger* – Averages roughly 95 calories per ounce.

- *Chicken Breast* – Averages 45 calories per serving over 14 items, with a range between 30 and 60 calories. Most items appeared in the 25 – 50-calorie range. A serving is usually one ounce, or a medium thickness slice.
- *Corned Beef* – Averages 56 calories per serving over four items, with a range between 40 and 71 calories. A serving is usually one ounce. Light or low fat variations run roughly 30 calories per serving.
- *Ham* – Averages 49 calories per serving over 29 items, with a range between 30 and 82 calories. Most items appeared in the 25 – 50 calorie range. A serving is usually one ounce, or one medium thickness slice.
- *Ham, Turkey* – Averages 31 calories per ounce over five items, with a range between 23 and 35 calories. A medium thickness slice is usually equivalent to one ounce.
- *Liverwurst* – Averages approximately 90 calories per ounce.
- *Pastrami* – Full beef is 98 calories per ounce, light varieties average around 40 calories per ounce.
- *Pepperoni* – Averages 70 calories per ounce.
- *Roast Beef* – Averages approximately 30 calories per ounce.
- *Salami, Beef and Pork* – Averages 90 calories per one-ounce serving over 30 items, with a range between 59 and 119 calories per ounce. Most items appeared in the 110-calorie range.
- *Salami, Turkey* – Averages 49 calories per ounce.
- *Sausage, Chicken* – Averages 58 calories per one-ounce serving over 10 items, with a range between 29 and 88 calories. Most items appeared in the 50 – 60 calorie range.
- *Sausage, Pork* – Averages 88 calories per ounce over 30 items, with a range between 46 and 113 calories. Most items appeared in the 90 – 100 calorie range.
- *Sausage, Turkey* – Averages 58 calories per one-ounce serving over 10 items, with a range between 29 and 88 calories. Most items appeared in the 50 – 60-calorie range.
- *Turkey* - Averages approximately 25 calories per ounce.

OILS

Corn Oil, Olive Oil, Peanut Oil etc. all run 120 calories per tablespoon.

|SALAD DRESSING/TOPPINGS

Bacon
Averages 127 calories per serving over four items, with a range between 80 and 150 calories. Most items appeared in the 130-calorie range. A serving is usually two tablespoons. Light varieties range less than 60 calories per serving.

Blue Cheese
Averages 144 calories per serving over four items, with a range between 90 and 180 calories. Most items appeared in the 130 – 160-calorie range. A serving is usually two tablespoons. Light varieties average 53 calories per serving over nine items, with a range between 10 and 100 calories. Most items appeared in the 25 – 50-calorie range. *Tip: If you see green cheese and you're not on the moon, don't eat it.*

Buttermilk
Averages 170 calories per serving over seven items, with a range between 150 and 180 calories. Most items appeared in the 130 – 160-calorie range. A serving is usually two tablespoons. Light varieties range roughly 90 calories per serving.

Caesar
Averages 145 calories per serving over 13 items, with a range between 100 and 190 calories. Most items appeared in the 130 – 160-calorie range. A serving is usually two tablespoons. Light varieties run roughly 50 calories per serving.

French
Averages 140 calories per serving, with light varieties averaging 60 calories per serving. A serving is usually two tablespoons.

Coleslaw
Averages 150 calories per serving, with light varieties averaging 50 calories per serving. A serving is usually two tablespoons.

Cucumber
Averages 150 calories per serving, with light varieties averaging 60 calories per serving. A serving is usually two tablespoons.

Garlic

Averages 137 calories per two-tablespoon serving over four items, with a range between 110 and 160 calories. Most items appeared in the 130 – 160-calorie range.

Honey Dijon, Honey Mustard, Honey Ranch

Averages 144 calories per serving over 10 items, with a range between 100 and 160 calories. Most items appeared in the 130 – 160-calorie range. A serving is usually two tablespoons. Light varieties average 45 calories per serving over 15 items, with a range between 15 and 80 calories. Most items appeared in the 25 – 50-calorie range.

Italian

Averages 123 calories per two tablespoon serving over 24 items, with a range between 90 and 180 calories. Most items appeared in the 100 – 110-calorie range. Light varieties average 31 calories per serving over 27 items, with a range between 5 and 90 calories. Most items appeared in the 25-calorie range.

Parmesan

Averages 160 calories per serving over four items, with a range between 140 and 180 calories. Most items appeared in the 130 – 160-calorie range. A serving is usually two tablespoons. Light varieties average 45 calories per serving.

Ranch

Averages 160 calories per serving over 21 items, with a range between 120 and 190 calories. Most items appeared in the 130 – 160-calorie range. A serving is usually two tablespoons. Light varieties average 52 calories per serving over 22 items, with a range between 5 and 110 calories. Most items appeared in the 25 – 50-calorie range.

Vinegar and Oil

Averages 120 calories per serving. A serving is usually two tablespoons.

Russian

Averages 127 calories per serving over four items, with a range between 110 and 150 calories. Most items appeared in the 110 – 130-calorie range. A serving is usually two tablespoons. Light varieties average 45 calories per serving.

Thousand Island

Averages 140 calories per serving over seven items, with a range between 100 and 240 calories. Most items appeared in the 130 – 160-calorie range. A serving is usually two tablespoons. Light varieties average 47 calories per serving over eight items, with a range between 35 and 70 calories. Most items appeared in the 25 – 50-calorie range.

Salad Toppings

Run around the 30 calories per serving range. This includes bacon bits and things of this type. It does not include croutons. Servings are usually one teaspoon.
  ❖ *Croutons – Aahh the lonely crouton,* standing by itself at 30
    calories for two tablespoons, or about nine croutons.

|SAUCES

Barbecue Sauce

Averages 51 calories per serving over 64 items, with a range between 20 and 60 calories. Most items appeared in the 50 - 60-calorie range. A serving is usually two tablespoons.

Chili Sauce

Runs roughly 15 – 20 calories per tablespoon, except hot dog chili sauce, which runs in the 100 calories per one-quarter cup range, because of the meat content.

Cocktail Sauce

Runs in the 60 calories per one-quarter cup serving with at least one brand as high as 100 calories per serving.

Enchilada Sauce

Runs around 25 calories per one-quarter cup. *(muy bueno)*

Honey

Averages 60 calories per tablespoon.

Horseradish
Averages eight calories per serving over 13 items, with a range between 0 and 25 calories. Most items appeared in the 10-calorie range. A serving is usually one teaspoon to one tablespoon.

Hot Sauce
Zero, zip, nada, no calories.

Miscellaneous Creamy Type Sauces
Including items like a la king, various cooking sauces, and béarnaise sauce. Averages 116 calories per serving over 44 items, with a range between 50 and 280 calories. Most items appeared in the 130 – 160-calorie range. A serving is usually one-half cup, or 8 tablespoons. Higher fat sauces tend to run to the higher end of the range. Light or low fat varieties average 22 calories per serving over 16 items, with a range between 5 and 50 calories. Most items appeared in the 25-calorie range. A serving is usually one-half cup.

Pasta Sauce
❖ *Alfredo Sauces* – Average 262 calories per serving over seven items, with a range between 110 and 400 calories. Values clustered in the 300-calorie range. A serving is usually one-half cup.
❖ *Tomato Based Sauce* – Averages 85 calories per serving over 120 items, with a range between 30 and 180 calories. Items clustered most frequently in the in the 60-calorie range. If the sauce has ingredients like meat or cheese, it tends to have more calories. Also beware of sauces with a high oil content, which can go over 600 calories per serving. (y*ikes, keep your cardiologist on speed dial if you eat this a lot)* Light versions can run in the 30 to 50-calorie range. A serving is usually one-half cup. **READ LABELS!**

Pesto Sauce
Averages 240 calories per serving over three items, with a range between 190 and 320 calories. A serving is usually one-quarter cup. There are also low fat mixes that are as low as 15 calories per serving.

Pizza Sauce
Averages 39 calories per serving over 18 items, with a range between 25 and 70 calories. Most items appeared in the 40-calorie range. A serving is usually one-quarter cup.

Relish
Averages 14 calories per serving over 15 items, with a range between 5 and 20 calories. A serving is usually one tablespoon.

Salsa and Picante Sauce
Runs approximately in the 10 – 15 calories per two tablespoons range.

Soy Sauce
Averages 10 calories per serving. A serving is *soytainly* one tablespoon, *nyuk nyuk.*

Steak Sauce
Averages 12 calories per one-tablespoon serving over nine items, with a range between 6 and 20 calories.

Stir Fry Sauce
Averages 19 calories per one-tablespoon serving over eight items, with a range between 9 and 40 calories.

Sweet and Sour Sauce
Does anybody else see the dichotomy in this name? Averages 62 calories per two-tablespoon serving over seven items, with a range between 35 and 80 calories.

Syrups and Toppings
Averages 121 calories per serving over 42 items, with a range between 50 and 220 calories. Most items appeared in the 110 – 130-calorie range. A serving is usually two tablespoons. Light varieties average 50 calories per serving over 11 items, with a range between 25 and 70 calories. Most items appeared in the 25 – 50-calorie range. A serving is usually two tablespoons.

Taco Sauce
Averages five calories per serving over eight items. A serving is usually one tablespoon.

Tahini
If you want to be teeny, go light on Tahini. Averages 145 calories per serving over six items, with a range between 80 and 200 calories. Most items, however, appeared in the 160 – 190-calorie range. A serving is usually two tablespoons.

Tartar Sauce
Averages 122 calories per serving over five items, with a range between 80 and 150 calories. A serving is usually two tablespoons. Light varieties run between 25 and 60.

Tomato Paste
Averages 30 calories per serving over eight items. A serving is usually two tablespoons.

Tomato Sauce
Averages 24 calories per serving over 27 items, with a range between 15 and 40 calories. Most items appeared in the 1 – 25-calorie range. A serving is usually one-quarter cup.

Worcestershire Sauce
Averages 0 to 8 calories. A serving is usually a tablespoon. *It took more energy to type "Worcestershire" than is in this stuff.*

SEAFOOD

Canned
- ❖ *Caviar* – When packed in olive oil, it runs 25 calories per tablespoon.
- ❖ *Clams* – Run between 15 and 30 calories per ounce, or between 30 and 60 per one-quarter cup for canned. *Just a note, bread and fry these suckers and they run 392 calories for a 3.5 ounce serving, or 112 calories per ounce.*
- ❖ *Cod* – Averages approximately 23 calories per ounce, or 189 calories per fillet for plain cod.
- ❖ *Crab* – Averages approximately 28 calories per ounce, or 182 calories per 6.5-oz can.
- ❖ *Lobster* – Averages roughly 83 calories an ounce for typical

cooked lobster.

- ❖ *Mackerel* – Averages approximately 60 calories per ounce, or 230 calories per fillet.
- ❖ *Mussels* – Averages 150 calories for a three-ounce serving.
- ❖ *Oysters* – Averages around 100 calories for a two-ounce serving.
- ❖ *Salmon* – Averages 90 calories per serving over 12 items, with a range between 60 and 110 calories. Most items appeared in the 90-calorie range. A serving is considered two and one-half ounces, so 36 – 44 calories per ounce.
- ❖ *Sardines* – Average 217 calories per serving over nine items, with a range between 120 and 290 calories. A serving is one can. The bulk of the calories seem to come from the way the fish is packed. Sardines usually come packed in oil. There are low calorie variants packed in sauce that are lower in fat and calories.
- ❖ *Scallops* – Average 35 calories per large item, or about 10 – 15 calories per small item.
- ❖ *Shrimp* - Runs between 25 and 30 calories per ounce.
- ❖ *Tuna* – In oil, averages 108 calories over nine items for a two-ounce serving. Most items fell into the 110-calorie per serving range, with a high of 160 calories and a low of 80 calories.
- ❖ *Tuna* – In water, averages 64 calories over 14 items for a two-ounce serving. Most items fell into the 60-calorie per serving range with a high of 80 calories and a low of 60 calories.

Freshwater and Saltwater Fish
Unless otherwise stated, all values are for broiled, grilled or baked items.
- ❖ *Ahi Tuna* – 90 calories / three-ounce serving
- ❖ *Anchovy* – 110 calories / three-ounce serving
- ❖ *Bass*– 120 calories / three-ounce serving
- ❖ *Bluefish* – 140 calories / three-ounce serving
- ❖ *Catfish, channel* – 130 calories / three-ounce serving
- ❖ *Caviar* – 210 calories / three-ounce serving
- ❖ *Cod* – 90 calories / three-ounce serving
- ❖ *Dolphinfish* – 90 calories / three-ounce serving
- ❖ *Flounder* – 100 calories / three-ounce serving
- ❖ *Haddock* – 96 calories / three-ounce serving
- ❖ *Halibut* – 120 calories / three-ounce serving
- ❖ *Herring, Atlantic* – 170 calories / three-ounce serving
- ❖ *Herring, Pacific* – 220 calories / three-ounce serving

- ❖ *Mackerel* – 220 calories / three-ounce serving
- ❖ *Monkfish* – 80 calories / three-ounce serving
- ❖ *Mullet* – 130 calories / three-ounce serving
- ❖ *Ocean Perch* – 100 calories / three-ounce serving
- ❖ *Orange Roughy* – 80 calories / three-ounce serving
- ❖ *Pike, northern* – 100 calories / three-ounce serving
- ❖ *Salmon, pink* – 130 calories / three-ounce serving
- ❖ *Sea Bass* - 110 calories / three-ounce serving
- ❖ *Sea Trout* – 110 calories / three-ounce serving
- ❖ *Shad, American* – 210 calories / three-ounce serving
- ❖ *Swordfish* – 130 calories / three-ounce serving
- ❖ *Trout* – 160 calories / three-ounce serving
- ❖ *Tuna, bluefin* – 160 calories / three-ounce serving
- ❖ *Tuna* – 120 calories / three-ounce serving
- ❖ *Walleye* – 100 calories / three-ounce serving
- ❖ *Whitefish* – 150 calories / three-ounce serving

Shellfish

Unless otherwise stated, all values are for broiled, grilled or baked items without shell.

- ❖ *Abalone* – 90 calories / three-ounce serving
- ❖ *Clams* – 60 calories / three-ounce serving
- ❖ *Clams, steamed* - 130 calories/ three-ounce serving
- ❖ *Crab* – 90 calories / three-ounce serving
- ❖ *Crab, cake* – 130 calories / three-ounce serving
- ❖ *Lobster* – 100 calories / three-ounce serving
- ❖ *Octopus* – 140 calories / three-ounce serving
- ❖ *Oysters* – 70 calories / three-ounce serving
- ❖ *Scallop* – 150 calories / three-ounce serving
- ❖ *Shrimp* – 110 calories / three-ounce serving
- ❖ *Squid* – 80 calories / three-ounce serving

|SNACKS

Chips

Average 144 calories per one-ounce serving over 115 items, with a range between 70 and 240 calories. Most items appeared in the 150-calorie range.

Popcorn
Runs approximately 31 calories per cup for air-popped, and 55 calories per cup for oil-popped. When you're at the movies, ask how many cups are in the mega tubs they sell. Could save your weight loss efforts.

Pretzels
Run around 110 calories per ounce.

Nuts
Mostly run in the 170 – 180-calorie per ounce range. Pecans run in the 190-calories per ounce range.

Seeds
Average 134 calories per one-ounce serving over 10 items, with a range between 25 and 170 calories. Most items appeared in the 160-calorie range.

|SPREADS

Jams, Jellies and Fruit Spreads
Not to be confused with "Jelly's Last Jam," which, like most musicals, contains no calories. This averages 37 calories per serving over 14 items, with a range between 20 and 50 calories. Most items appeared in the 40-calorie range. A serving is one tablespoon.

Peanut Butter and Nut Spreads
Averages 184 calories per serving over 32 items, with a range between 150 and 200 calories. Most items appeared in the 190-calorie range. A serving is two tablespoons.

Ketchup
Averages 15 calories per serving over six items, with a range between 10 and 25 calories. Most items appeared in the 15-calorie range. A serving is usually one tablespoon.

Marinades
Average 20 calories per serving over 11 items, with a range between 10 and 40 calories. Most items appeared in the 20-calorie range. A serving is usually one tablespoon.

Mayonnaise and Mayonnaise Type Dressing
Averages 100 calories per serving for regular mayonnaise, light mayonnaise averages 35 over eight items, with a range between 25 and 50, fat free gets down into the 10 – 15-calorie range, and Miracle Whip® runs 70 calories. A serving is usually one tablespoon.

Mustard
Runs between 0 and 10 calories for approximately one teaspoon.

| VEGETABLES, CANNED

❖ *Artichoke Hearts* – Run approximately 17 calories per item.
❖ *Asparagus* – Run roughly 20 calories for a one-half cup serving.
❖ *Bamboo Shoots* – These run 15 calories per ounce. *No caloric value if you just put them under your fingernails. Note to self: need to quit watching old war movies.*
❖ *Beans* – Average 122 calories per serving over 181 items, with a range between 80 and 350 calories. The greatest number of items appeared in the 120 – 130-calorie range. A serving here is usually one-half cup. *You should probably avoid these on a first date; 'nuff said.* These values are for starchy beans, Green Beans, on the other hand, only average roughly 25 calories per one-half cup. *So remember, if you want to lose weight, don't be a weenie, keep your beans mostly greenie.*
❖ *Beets* – Average 51 calories per one-half cup serving over 10 items, with a range between 35 and 90 calories. Most items appeared in the 40-calorie range. *Even if you eat a lot of these, there's really no reason to "beet" yourself up over it.*
❖ *Carrots* – Run about 35 calories for a one-half cup serving.
❖ *Corn* – Runs roughly 70 calories per one-third cup.
❖ *Cream Corn* – Runs roughly 100 – 110 calories per one-half cup.
❖ *Mushrooms* – Average 34 calories per one-half cup serving over 12 items, with a range between 25 and 80 calories.
❖ *Onions* – Average around 40 calories per one-half cup.
❖ *Peas* – Average 82 calories per one-half cup serving over 29 items, with a range between 50 and 120 calories. Most items appeared in the 60-calorie range.

❖ *Peppers* – Usually land in the 10 – 20-calorie per item range, fried go into the 60 range.

❖ *Potato* – Averages 77 calories for one-half to two-thirds cup.

❖ *Sauerkraut* – Averages 33 calories per one-half cup serving over five items, with a range between 10 and 60 calories. Most items appeared in the 50-calorie range.

❖ *Spinach* – Averages 19 calories per three and a half ounce serving over seven items, with a range between 30 and 45 calories.

❖ *Squash – Even if you squeeze it really hard*, it averages 36 calories per one-cup serving.

❖ *Succotash* – Averages 115 calories per 3.5-ounce serving.

❖ *Sweet Potatoes* – Average 182 calories per one-half cup serving over five items, with a range between 120 and 210 calories. Most items appeared in the 200-calorie range.

❖ *Tomatoes* – Average 29 calories per serving over 43 items, with a range between 20 and 45 calories. A serving is usually considered one-half cup.

❖ *Turnip Greens* – Average 27 calories per one-half cup.

❖ *Vegetables, mixed* – Run roughly 40 calories per one-half cup.

❖ *Water Chestnuts* – Average 15 calories per one-half cup.

❖ *Yams* – Average 160 calories per two-thirds cup.

❖ *Zucchini* – Averages 35 calories per one-half cup.

| VEGETABLES, FROZEN

❖ *Artichokes* – 40 calories per one-half cup

❖ *Asparagus* – 25 calories per one-half cup

❖ *Beans* – 115 calories per one-half cup

❖ *Broccoli* – 25 calories per one-half cup

❖ *Brussels Sprouts* – 35 calories per one-half cup

❖ *Carrots* – 35 calories per one-half cup

❖ *Cauliflower* – 25 calories per one-half cup

❖ *Collards* – 30 calories per one-half cup

❖ *Corn* – 70 calories per one-half cup

❖ *Mustard Greens* – 15 calories per one-half cup

❖ *Onions* – 20 calories per one-half cup

❖ *Peas* – 70 calories per one-half cup

❖ *Peppers* – 20 calories per one-half cup

❖ *Potatoes, mashed* – 80 calories per one-half cup
❖ *Spinach* – 30 calories per one-half cup
❖ *Squash* – 15 calories per one-half cup
❖ *Succotash* – 70 calories per one-half cup
❖ *Sweet Potato* – 90 calories per one-half cup
❖ *Turnip Greens* – 20 calories per one-half cup

😊 Here's a tip. You can sum up the frozen vegetables by saying that starchy veggies are approximately 100 calories per one-half cup, the rest fall into the 25 – 50-calorie range. *By now, you should have it down pat that butter is 35 calories per those little square things. Hmmm, now what are they called? Anyway, make sure to add the butter to your calorie total.*

VEGETABLES, RAW

❖ *Artichoke* – 60 calories / medium item
❖ *Asparagus* – 30 calories / cup
❖ *Bean, fava* – 40 calories / one-half cup
❖ *Bean green* – 15 calories / one-half cup
❖ *Bean, Lima* – 90 calories / one-half cup
❖ *Bean, yellow* – 15 calories / one-half cup
❖ *Beet* – 30 calories / one-half cup
❖ *Broccoli* – 10 calories / one-half cup
❖ *Cabbage* – 20 calories / cup
❖ *Cabbage, red* – 20 calories / cup
❖ *Carrot* – 25 calories / one-half cup
❖ *Cauliflower* – five calories / one-half cup
❖ *Celery* – five calories / stalk *(look who stalking now)*
❖ *Collard* – 10 calories / cup
❖ *Corn* – 70 calories / one-half cup
❖ *Eggplant* – five calories / one-half cup *(no need for a chicken if you've got one of these)*
❖ *Endive* – 10 calories / cup
❖ *Garlic* – zero calories / clove *(this explains its new popularity as chewing gum, HAHA just jesting... Was an explanation really necessary here?)*
❖ *Kale* – 35 calories / cup
❖ *Leek* – 35 calories / one-half cup

- *Lettuce* – 10 to 20 calories / one-half cup
- *Mushroom* – 10 calories / one-half cup
- *Okra* – 20 calories / one-half cup
- *Onion* – 30 calories / one-half cup
- *Pea, green* – 60 calories / one-half cup
- *Pea, snow* – 35 calories / one-half cup
- *Potato, baked* – 220 calories / item with skin
- *Potato, baked* – 120 calories / cup without skin
- *Pumpkin* – 10 calories / one-half cup
- *Spinach* – 15 calories / cup
- *Squash* – 31 calories / medium sized item
- *Succotash* – 110 calories / one-half cup
- *Sweet Potato* – 100 calories / one-half cup, with skin (*name refers to flavor, not disposition*)
- *Tomato, green* – 30 calories / item (*no, they're not this color because they envy their red cousins*)
- *Tomato, red* – 25 calories / item (*no, they're not this color because they're embarrassed by their green cousins*)
- *Turnip* – 20 calories / one-half cup
- *Yam* – 177 calories / cup

You might notice that raw veggies are much lower, calorically, than frozen. This may be due to additives in the frozen food, not sure.   READ LABELS!!!

|VENERABLE BAR FOODS

The word "venerable" was chosen here so that these fun foods would be the last on the list; thus leaving the gentle reader with a pleasant impression while maintaining a, time-honored, somewhat alphabetical order.

Cheeseburger
Approximately 550 calories for a four-ounce burger with roll.

Cheese steak
Really depends on a lot of factors, but a typical six to eight-inch sandwich will cost somewhere around 700 – 1000 calories. *Great candidate to split*

with a significant other, friend, co-worker, brother, sister, mom, dad, cousins...

Chicken Wings
- ❖ Bone in – Average 70 calories per wing depending on what sauce is on it. Be careful, sauces can really jack up this value.
- ❖ Boneless – Average 90 calories per wing depending on what sauce is on it.

Clams Breaded and Fried
Run 392 calories for a 3.5-ounce serving, or 112 calories per ounce.

Deviled Eggs
Really dependent on the amount of mayonnaise and egg yolk used, but typically in the 65-calorie range for half an egg.

French Fries
Approximately 220 calories per 100 gram or 3.5 ounce individual serving. Think the size of a small fast food bag of fries.

French Fries with Cheese
Approximately 270 – 300 calories per 100 gram or 3.5 ounce individual serving. Think the size of a small fast food bag of fries.

Hamburger
Approximately 480 - 490 calories for a four-ounce burger and roll.

Jalapeno Bites, Poppers, Snacks
Approximately 350 calories for a four-ounce serving. You might want to share this.

Mozzarella Stick
One three-inch long stick with a diameter of roughly one-half inch is approximately 70 – 90 calories per item.

Mushrooms, Stuffed
Calories for stuffed mushrooms depend on what's stuffing them. They can be as low as 35 per mushroom to over 100 calories per mushroom. The

variety most commonly seen in restaurants and bars seems to be stuffed with crabmeat, and these are roughly 50 calories per mushroom.

Nachos
Ranges from 90 – 100 calories per nacho with cheese and jalapeno pepper.

Olives
Usually run about 25 calories per three olives.

Pickles
Average 16 calories per serving over 44 items, with a range between 5 and 45 calories. A serving here is usually one spear. Sweet pickles run toward the 45-calorie range per serving.

Pizza
Roughly 275 calories per typical slice, thin crust runs approximately 200 calories per slice, or approximately two-thirds as much as regular crust.

Potato Skins
Average 75 calories per item with cheese and bacon.

Roast Beef Sandwich
Roughly 300 – 350 calories for small sandwich, add about 60 – 75 calories for cheese. Add 75 – 100 calories for mayonnaise.

After you use this list, or the other sources of dietary data that are available, you should find that you develop your own, "down and dirty," quick reference list. Such a list can be invaluable as you ease your way into a calorically-aware lifestyle.

In the storyline, I have used examples revolving mostly around restaurant eating, because I wanted to show that this approach could hold up in the most challenging situations. If you are someone who primarily eats at home, and buys most of your food from a supermarket, this approach is even easier because most things are labeled, and the choices are virtually limitless. This also makes it a cinch to add up the ingredients in a given recipe and create your own personalized calorie index.

Experience teaches that there will always be people who feel that calorie counting is a headache, and of course, they are entitled to that opinion. This author prefers to look at it as a tradeoff. If you trade the time and minor inconvenience to monitor your caloric intake, you earn the ability to eat anything you want, not diet everyday, and maintain a good body weight. Sounds like time well spent to us. Since there is no motivational talk as effective as success, the final words in this section are: just do it!

To Phil's Relief, Grunting And Groaning Is Strictly Optional

It's 9:00 AM on a sterling Saturday in late May. The countryside near Gloria's home is dressed in its full spring regalia featuring trees gravid with blossoms, and impossibly green foliage. Gloria and Phil have been dating for roughly two months. Phil has lost twelve pounds and is amazed by how easy it is to stick to his weekly mini-diet, as he likes to call it.

Gloria is puttering around her kitchen while she waits for him to arrive. Her heart is light and she smiles when she sees him walking up her driveway. He is wearing jeans, jogging shoes, a tee shirt and a light jacket, perfect for the activity Gloria has planned. It is a full-calorie day for both of them, and she knows Phil is looking forward to a nice breakfast at a quaint local bistro they have been frequenting.

Just as Phil raises his hand to knock on her door, she opens it and before he can drop his arm, she slips under it and hugs him. While he is fumbling for words, she quickly pushes her door shut, takes his hand and begins to walk toward the street. Phil stumbles after her, wearing a nonplussed look. Before he can fully regain his balance, she turns back to look at him and says, "C'mon, guy, I can only drag you so far."

Seeing the impish twinkle in her eyes, he knows this means he is about to be introduced to something new. Phil, like most guys, is not necessarily crazy about "new" things, and says so. "OK, Gloria, I know that look. What are we doing?"

Sidestepping the mild agitation in his voice she answers, "I'm glad you said 'we' Phil. It makes me feel like we're a team, like we have a bond."

Eyes narrowing with doubt, he rejoins, "Of course I too like the idea of us being a team," making the 'quote' gesture with his fingers, "but I'm getting the sneaking suspicion that I'm being roped into something, aahh, new."

"Oh, just c'mon this way, I want to show you something," she says playfully, as she jerks him toward the road.

At that time, Gloria lived in a semi-rural area where the roads tended to be narrow and the hills steep. Her street was no exception and the incline they had to climb caused Phil to visibly huff a bit, despite his best efforts to hide it. After only a few minutes, though, they took a hard left down a narrow, overgrown path, steep enough to require grabbing overhanging branches for balance. After a few yards, Gloria led Phil to the right along a much wider intersecting trail that ran alongside a noisy, boulder-strewn creek. This was the first time they had been so alone, and Phil nervously joked about her wanting to get him in the woods. Gloria smiled devilishly, and then she reached for his hand. For almost a half-hour they walked, enmeshed in light conversation punctuated by the occasional birdsong and the wind as it rustled the treetops. Finally, they came upon a meadow with a single, huge oak tree standing in the middle, as though it had pushed all the other trees aside.

Gloria led Phil to the base of the tree and said they should rest there. She then sat down, her back against the tree. Phil sat on the ground opposite her. For many moments neither one broke the blessed silence. They just held each other's hands while alternately drinking in the natural beauty that surrounded them, and stealing the occasional glance into each other's soul. After a while, Phil, fidgeting a bit and seeming a little nervous, tried to engage Gloria in small talk. She placed her fingers against his lips and locked his gaze with her own. "This is where Hugh and I used to come." Phil smiled a sad smile, apparently not knowing how to feel or respond to this. Sensing his misunderstanding, she squeezed both his hands, and said, "I want to make new memories now." Here, they kissed for the first time. It was a good first kiss, soft and gentle, their lips barely brushing against each other, but the flood of feeling was enough to tell them both that this was the right time.

The walk back was characterized by lively conversation, and the handholding was replaced by arms around waists, shoulders etc. It was as though they had just discovered each other, nay, just discovered the only other man and woman in existence. Phil didn't really understand this yet, but Gloria did. She knew she was truly falling in love, and at the moment she was happy. She knew she would cry later.

Phil and Gloria never made it to their little bistro for breakfast. As it happened, they "fell into" an activity that obviated all interest in food until the early evening. It wasn't until they were driving to dinner that the conversation returned to dieting. Gloria was smiling a cat-that-caught-the-canary-smile when she said, "I have another surprise for you, Phil."

"I don't know if I can take another surprise today."

She laughed and said, "Oh, I'm quite sure you'll like this one, maybe not as much as the last one, but..." he looked at her expectantly and she continued, "You know, everything we did today can be considered exercise." She paused for a minute when she noticed the corners of his lips beginning to curl upward. She continued, "You probably burned, and this is a conservative estimate, an extra 300 calories today, which means you can have an extra one or two of those imported beers you like so much."

"Well that shoots the "no pain, no gain" axiom in the umm," he hesitated and decided to keep it clean, "foot." They both snickered and Gloria noticed Phil turned red at his own joke. The dinner that finally ensued was savored.

As the days progressed, Gloria introduced Phil to more ways to burn calories and reinforced the idea that exercise did not have to be an all or none proposition that left one feeling worse instead of better. Phil, not being a very physical male, had always thought that meaningful exercise was something that was beyond him. He had always felt he just wasn't capable, because of desire and, or genetics, of following a regimen that would produce any benefit. Gloria had now taught him that exercise was a tool that could be used to accomplish "his" goals, however grand or modest they might be. Thanks to her, Phil is now armed with the knowledge that the amount and intensity of the work is directly related to what he wants to achieve.

Over the rest of this chapter, I will highlight some basic principles of exercise, and how to use it to maintain muscle tissue for long-term weight loss. If I do my job correctly, when you finish this chapter, you too should be imbued with the ability to design and implement your own exercise program based on your goals. Now, let's get started. ⇒⇒⇒⇒⇒⇒⇒⇒

Most of us have become desensitized to what was once considered foul language. It is quite common to hear all but the most heinous language on prime time television, and the vast majority of us don't even flinch. There is one word, though, that can still elicit paroxysms of disgust from even the most stoic among us, and that word is "exercise."

Before you go diving for the couch, let us just tell you that exercise does not have to mean grunting out set after set of squats, hours sweating in a spinning class, running wind sprints with the local high school football team, or herniating spinal discs in an aerobic dance class. If you like those things, then have at it, but be aware, they are not the only roads to a great body. For example, walking 30 minutes, five days per week will work wonders, especially if you have a sit-down job, and the only exercise you are presently doing consists of cringing in the face of approaching deadlines, or flinching as the boss flails some document about and browbeats you over some perceived insufficiency supported by said document. By the way, you can take solace in the fact that flinching burns more calories than flailing, so you, not your overwrought boss, will really get the last laugh. While there is no data to back up this assertion, we just know it's true because if there one iota of fairness in the universe, it should be. And speaking of truth, the truth is you can forget the entire preceding diatribe if you just remember these two principles: firstly, in order for an exercise program to work, you must do it consistently – so pick activities you like – and secondly, you must vary the routine frequently. Exactly how to vary your routine will be outlined in the next sections.

General Principles

To be perfectly honest, you can lose weight without exercise, at least short-term, but diet and exercise complement each other so well that one without the other is sort of like Garfunkel without Simon. You get the picture. Increasing your activity level is an important component of weight loss, because it helps increase your caloric debt. Remember, debt is something owed to somebody, and that somebody is you. That's right, activity increases the number of calories you owe yourself. Pretty neat concept, owing yourself food. Another no less important reason to exercise is that it helps to retain muscle tissue, which is critical to keeping your BMR at its highest.

There are two basic types of exercise: aerobic and anaerobic. Aerobic exercise uses large muscle groups repetitively for extended periods of time.

As the name implies, aerobic exercise uses a lot of oxygen. Examples of this type of exercise are: walking, running, cycling, aerobic dancing, and an array of machines designed for this purpose. Anaerobic exercise uses heavier resistance, i.e., heavier weight, or higher intensity. Higher intensity, in this case, means the exercise is performed faster and for a much shorter duration. For example, sprinting can be considered anaerobic, while jogging is aerobic. These are similar movements with different effects because of the different intensity and duration of each. If you don't believe this, look at the way a sprinter's legs are built versus a marathoner's legs: fast running versus slow running. Anaerobic exercise tends to use less oxygen than aerobic, and is often used to increase muscle size. Although anaerobic exercise does not tend to burn a lot of body fat while you are doing it, its ability to increase your BMR by increasing muscle size makes it at least as important as aerobic exercise for long-term weight management. Of course, there are many forms of anaerobic exercise besides sprinting. Chief among these are calisthenics like pushups, sit-ups, pull-ups etc, but the best example of this type of exercise is weight lifting, and the myriad machines that mimic this type of progressive resistance.

Before beginning any exercise program, it is wise to first decide what your goals for said program will be. For many people, this is easy and boils down to simply losing body fat and maintaining muscle tissue. Others may want to get a little more technical and focus on something more specific, like increasing muscle mass, enhancing flexibility or improving cardiovascular fitness, in addition to losing weight. Depending on what your goals are, you may focus on any of these areas, but a good fitness program will address all of these elements and utilize both anaerobic and aerobic exercise. In this chapter, I have highlighted some basic guidelines for each of these modes of exercise, and then put a few sample programs together, so you can get a good head start and see results quickly.

Before we get into the details, ladies, listen up! At the risk of sounding sexist, you do want to maintain muscle tissue! Muscle gives you your shape and, let's never forget, burns calories, so when you reach your goal weight, you will be able to eat more than hummingbird-sized portions and still maintain your goal weight long after the pages of this book have turned to dust.

Last, But Certainly Not Least, As With The Diet, You Should Not Start Any Exercise Program Without Your Doctor's OK. OK?

Progressive Resistance Exercise

Strictly speaking, progressive resistance exercise is a subset of anaerobic exercise, but in the real world, it is the most popular way that anaerobic training gets done. Progressive resistance exercise (PRE) refers to any exercise where you gradually increase the resistance you will push or pull against. This is done because, as you train, your body gets stronger. Your muscles will only adapt to the forces they must resist, so to keep them growing, you must raise the bar – forgive the pun – by increasing the resistance. Most commonly, this resistance is provided by free weights, but as mentioned previously, there are machines or apparatus that can also provide progressive resistance. These machines may use weights attached in some way, some form of elastic band, or compressed air to achieve this effect. The important fact to remember is that in order to improve muscle tone or size, we must constantly challenge the body to adapt to the changing environment we throw at it. Sound familiar? It should because it is the same concept we employ with the dietary aspect of this approach. Increasing resistance is only one way that we challenge the body, another very important way is to change the actual exercises we perform.

If you have access to a gym and you are comfortable with that atmosphere, increasing weight or resistance as needed should be a simple matter. Also, a good gym should have enough equipment to make varying your exercises easy. But wait, what if you don't belong to a gym? Maybe you can't afford it, or maybe you simply don't like that whole scene. No problem, you can put together a nice little program with a set of dumbbells and a little imagination. To help you with this, pictures have been provided with all the exercises mentioned. Study these carefully and read the captions, as proper form is essential to safety and effectiveness.

> **One Caveat: If You Are A Beginner, Or Unsure Of Proper Technique, It Is A Good Idea To Have Someone Familiar With The Proper Way To Perform Each Exercise Show You How To Do Them.**

PREs are an effective way to increase muscle strength, endurance, or both. Oops, let's define our terms. Endurance, for our purposes, will be defined as the ability to perform a movement, against resistance, a certain number of times. This is popularly thought of as toning. Strength refers to the ability to contract a muscle against heavier and heavier resistance, and, if done correctly, is accompanied by an increase in muscle size. Most PRE programs will produce some combination of the two.

A fairly accurate rule of thumb regarding PREs is that to add muscle size, and increase strength, you must lift as much weight as you can handle for five to six repetitions, **while maintaining proper form**. If your focus is more on toning, you must lift as much weight as you can handle for 15 to 20 repetitions, again, **while maintaining proper form**. One good way to employ these rules is to cycle them. By that I mean, focus on muscle size for a certain amount of time, perhaps two months, then focus on toning for a similar amount of time.

Aerobic Exercise

We have all seen the infomercials with the leotard-bedecked women and men dancing very energetically and demonstratively flailing their extremities to some infectiously upbeat music. They are led, more often than not, by a young, nubile instructor who has never had a weight problem and who seems to possess twice as much energy as any four members of the congregation. These instructors all seem to use the same folksy lingo, as they constantly refer to their audience as "gang" or "people" while exhorting them, with an almost religious fervor, to "Pick it up." This is, indeed, one form of aerobic exercise but thankfully, not the only one.

As mentioned before, aerobic exercise is any exercise that uses large muscle groups repeatedly and for extended periods of time. By extended periods of time, I mean ideally, 30 minutes or more, although it is perfectly OK to start with less. Walking, running, and biking are all good examples of this type of exercise.

Why 30 minutes, you might be wondering? From our experience, it seems that 30 minutes seems to be a good balance between burning a significant number of calories, and pushing the edge of psychological "burnout." Studies have also shown that when you first start doing aerobic exercise, you are mainly running on a substance called glycogen, which is a form of quick energy that is stored in the muscles and liver. Incidentally, glycogen requires water to be stored, and this property of glycogen storage can make it seem like a dieter has gained back one or two pounds in an inordinately short time. We will talk more about this in chapter six, the maintenance chapter.

As the exercise continues, provided it is done at a moderate pace, you gradually depend less on glycogen and more on your fat reserves for energy.

(an exact definition of moderate pace will be given in a minute) By the end of a 30-minute session of this type of exercise, you should be running mostly on body fat. If you want to exercise longer, that's fine and it will burn more calories, but be careful of physical and, the aforementioned, psychological "burnout."

The best way to explain psychological burnout is to refer to a principle espoused by body builders that recommends to "stay hungry." This basically means: don't overdo any one session so you don't destroy your motivation for the next workout. These are words by which to live.

If you are not used to any exercise at all, walking is probably the best place to start. I stated that walking for 30 minutes per day, five days per week will work wonders, but you might be thinking that you can't even do that much. This is not a problem. Believe it or not, starting with one minute on the first day and adding a minute on subsequent days is a great way to begin your sojourn to fitness. Think about it; if you do five sessions per week, after one month, you will be up to 20 minutes per session, and within six weeks, you will be at 30 minutes per session. Remember, weight loss is a marathon, not a sprint.

Even though the main purpose exercise serves in this book is sustainable weight loss, this tome would be less than complete if I did not point out that aerobic exercise can also be used to improve cardiovascular health. Although the types of programs to accomplish each of these goals have a lot of overlap, they are not identical. As you shall see, the difference is really a matter of intensity.

To extract maximum cardiovascular benefit from a workout, you must get your heart rate into what has been referred to as the target zone. According to the American Heart Association,[2] the target zone is 50 – 75 percent of your maximum heart rate. To find your <u>maximum</u> heart rate, simply subtract your age from 220. To find your <u>target</u> heart rate, you will multiply this number by somewhere between 0.5 and 0.75. So, for a typical sedentary 40-year-old man, the calculation goes like this: 220 minus 40 is 180. One hundred eighty times 0.5 is 90. This means that if he gets his heart rate into the 90 range for the duration of his aerobic workout, he will achieve a benefit to his heart and cardiovascular system. As he becomes fitter, he can gradually increase the multiplier until he is in the 0.75 range, in other words, he would multiply his maximum heart rate by 0.75, which in

---

[2] American Heart Association
http://www.justmove.org/myfitness/actarticles/acframes.cfm?Target=hartrates.html

his case is 180 X .75 or 135. **REMEMBER, THIS FORMULA ASSUMES NO PRE-EXISTING HEART DISEASE.**

A erobic exercise for maximum fat burning requires a slightly different set of numbers. The common wisdom indicates that to utilize the maximum amount of body fat during a given workout, the target heart rate zone is maximum heart rate times 0.60. So, to use the above 40-year-old man, we would say his ideal heart rate to burn body fat is 180 X .60, which is 108 beats per minute. You might think that higher would be better, but when you raise the heart rate much more than this, you start to tap into the anaerobic sources of energy, which tend to use more glycogen, instead of body fat. This is the definition of the "moderate pace" mentioned in the beginning of this section.

Incidentally, if you can't find your pulse, or have some other problem using this procedure, you can always fall back on another old rule of thumb that states: if you can talk without gasping while you are doing your workout, then you are probably not overdoing it. Be forewarned, if you use this little test while walking or running ALONE, you may garner more attention from your neighbors and the local gendarmerie than you might want, just a friendly little tip.

Putting Your Exercise Program Together

As mentioned before, this book is not a bodybuilding guide. Our focus is weight loss and preservation of muscle tissue during this process, so these recommendations will reflect this bias. There are many other ways to approach exercise, and your individual goals will dictate your actual approach.

A good starter program could include five days per week of aerobic exercise and two days per week of anaerobic exercise. The aerobic exercise can consist of simply getting out and taking a walk, and the anaerobic can be two sessions with dumbbells. (Ladies, this does not mean your male acquaintances, it means those small hand weights.)

The particulars of this program could look like this: Monday through Friday, walk for some period of time, say ten minutes. Monday and Thursday in addition to the walk do PREs, i.e., lift weights for 15 – 20 minutes. As your physical fitness improves, you could work this up to walking a half-hour per day for five days per week, and bump the PREs to one-half to three-quarter hour sessions.

With as few as two PRE workouts per week, you will begin to see changes in muscle size, strength, and endurance in as little as a month. Just like with the diet though, you will find that after doing the same routine for a while, the effectiveness of your program will diminish, or even stop. And, just like in dieting, you have reached a plateau, i.e., your body has learned to perform the tasks you put before it on fewer calories and without increasing muscle size. This is not the time to add to your exercise program. This is the time to change your program. There is a term called "muscle memory," which basically refers to the body's ability to learn to perform a certain movement or skill more efficiently. Works great if you want to become more skillful at something, but for our purposes, it slows the calorie burning and muscle building or preservation process. This may seem counterintuitive, but it is true. The better you get at something, the fewer calories you burn while doing it. And speaking of calories, if at all possible, try to coincide full DCN days with workouts. This will help with muscle preservation and even muscle growth.

Aerobic exercise follows the same principles, so if you are walking 30 minutes per day, after about 90 days, you may want to try jogging, or bicycling, or an elliptical trainer. Very often, you will find that when you change exercises, you will not be able to do the full 30 minutes. This is exactly what you want because the fact that you cannot do as much of the new exercise indicates that the body is now back to learning, and you should see the best weight loss during this phase.

Remember, pick activities that you like and that you are capable of doing. Jogging may not be your thing, but walking, elliptical training, stationary biking, and a ski machine will give you four activities you can use to make up a full year of training. In effect, you could use a sort of a seasonal approach where you could use a stationary bike during the winter, elliptical trainer during the spring, ski machine during the summer and walk during the fall. This agrees with the notion that exercise programs should be changed every 90 days. Varying the intensity of the exercises themselves is another way to keep the body guessing, so fast walking versus slow walking could also be employed to change things up, or carrying hand weights while walking could also increase the intensity and burn a few more calories. In the next section, I have included some basic exercise illustrations and routines that could be done at home with a minimum of equipment. The illustrations have been grouped with their respective routines.

SAMPLE WEIGHT LIFTING ROUTINES

Routine One

1- Shoulder Shrug – one to three sets of 10 repetitions

Shoulder Shrug

Start/End Position   Mid-Position

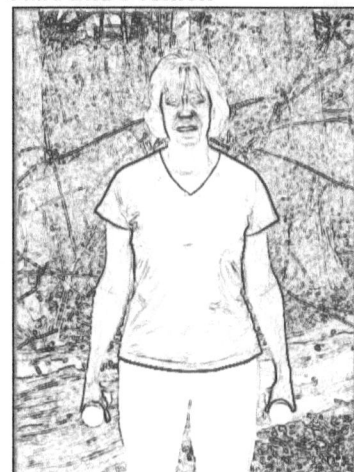
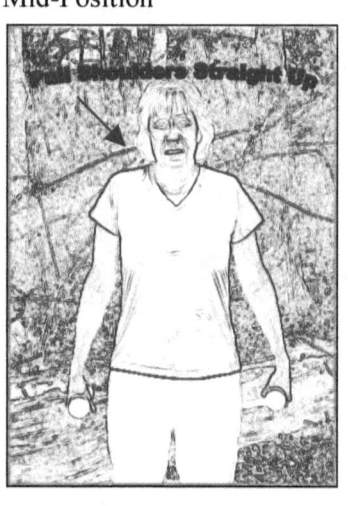

2- Shoulder Press – one to three sets of 10 repetitions

Shoulder Press

Start/End Position   Mid-Position

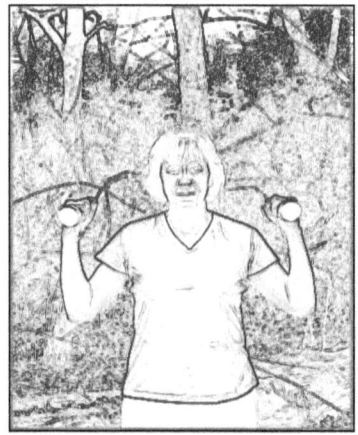
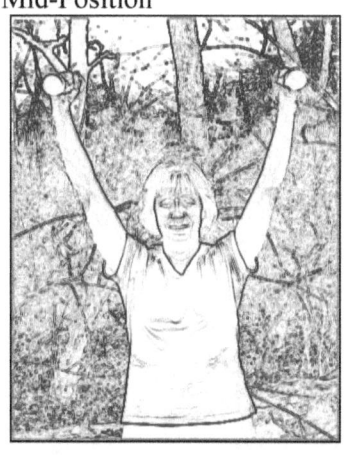

3-Arm Curl With Palms Up – one to three sets of 10 repetitions

Arm Curls With Palms Up

Start/End Position   Mid Position

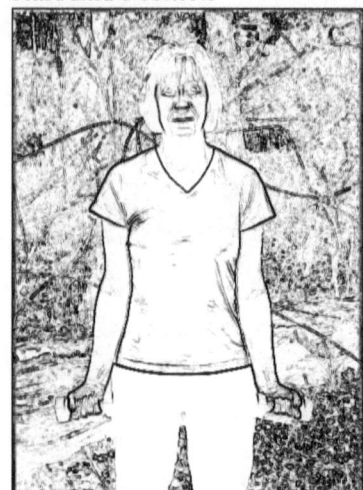 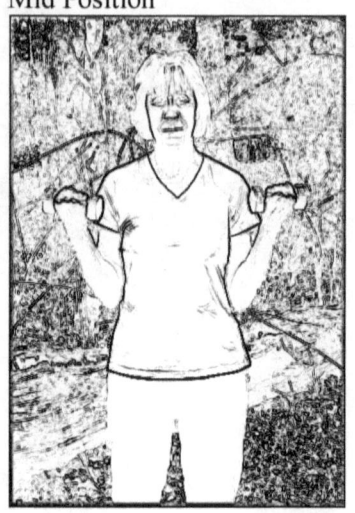

4-Arm Curl, Palms Down – one to three sets of 10 repetitions

Arm Curls Palms Down

Same as above, but with palms facing down.

5-Pushup Pivoting Off Of Knees With Hands Shoulder Width
– one to three sets of 10 repetitions

Pushup Pivoting Off Of Knees With Hands Shoulder Width

Start/End Position   Mid Position

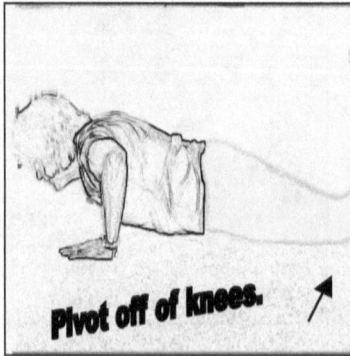 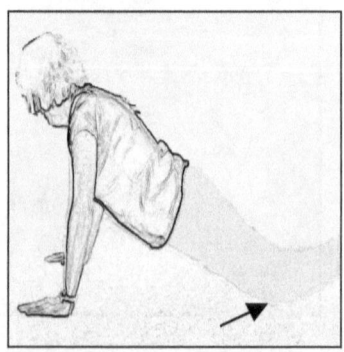

Pivot off of knees.

6-One Arm Dumbbell Row – one to three sets of 10 repetitions

One Arm Dumbbell Row

Start/End Position   Mid-Position

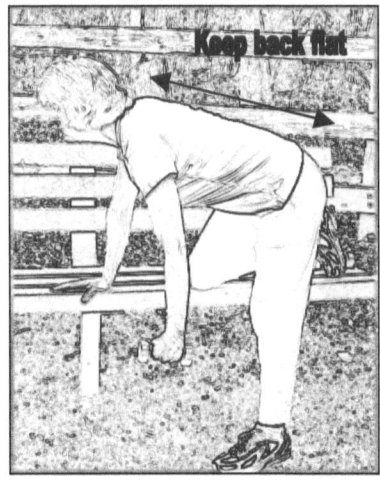
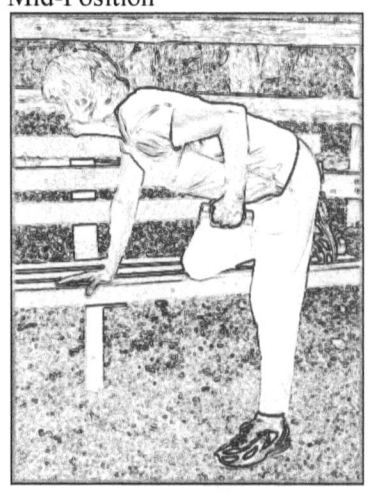

7-Squat/Clean – one to three sets of 10 repetitions

Squat/Clean

Start/End Position   Mid Position

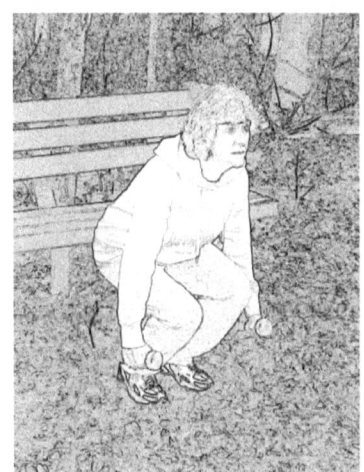
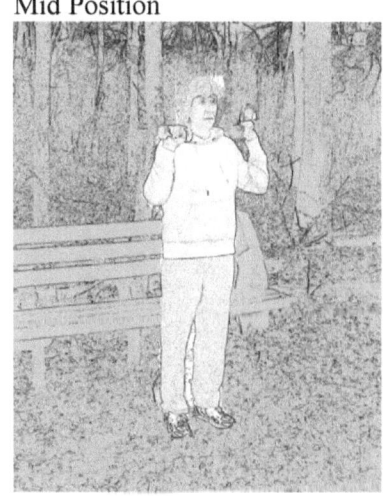

Use very light weight, keep your head up so as to keep your back straight. Start in squat position and raise the dumbbells to shoulder height as you stand. **If you have any history of back injury, back pain or previous leg pain, especially extending from the back, or if you feel back pain when doing it, do not do this exercise.**

8-Abdominal Crunch– one to three sets of 10 repetitions

Abdominal Crunch

Start/End Position   Mid-Position

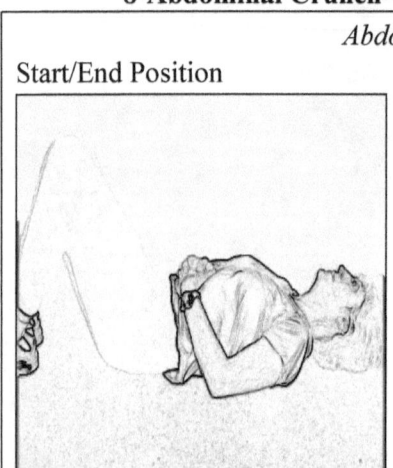
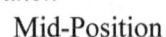
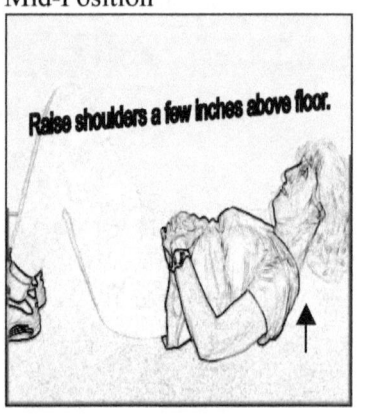

Raise shoulders a few inches above floor.

9-Half Squat – one to three sets of 10 repetitions (notice dumbbells in each hand to increase resistance)

Squat- Half/Full

Start/End Position   Mid-Position

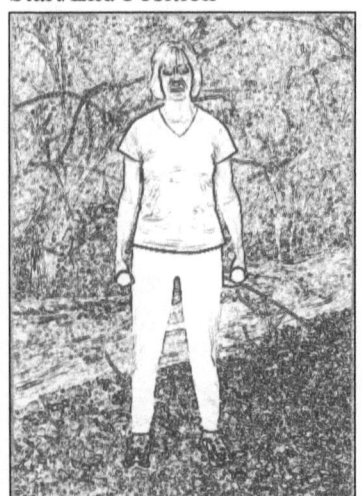
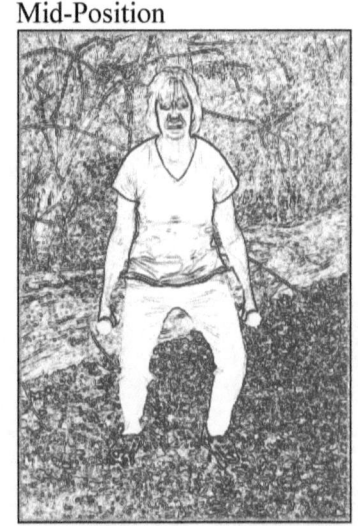

Here we illustrate the <u>half-squat</u> with knees bent to approx 45 degrees in the mid-position. To do the <u>Full squat</u> you would bend to 90 degrees in the mid-position, or about twice as far. Keep back straight.

10-Standing Leg Curl – one to three sets of 10 repetitions (ankle
weights or heavy shoes can be used for resistance)

Standing Leg Curl

Start/End Position   Mid-Position

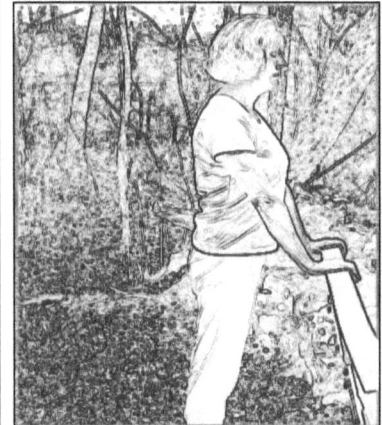 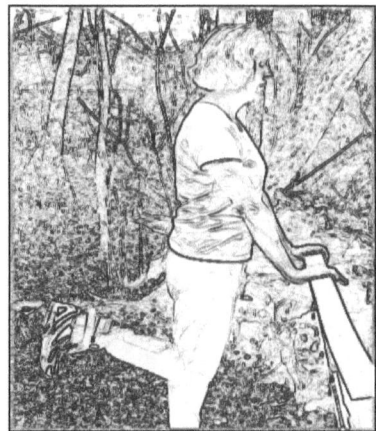

<u>Prone Leg Curl</u> is done the same way, but instead of standing, you are lying
on your stomach and bending your knee.

11-Standing Calf Raise (toes forward) – one to three sets of 10 repetitions

Standing Calf Raise

Start/End Position   Mid-Position

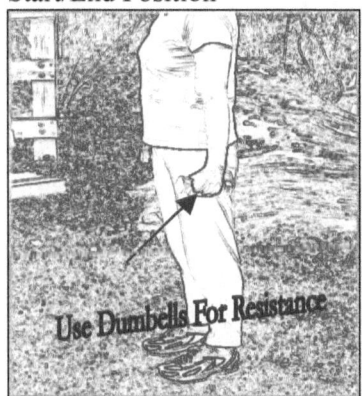 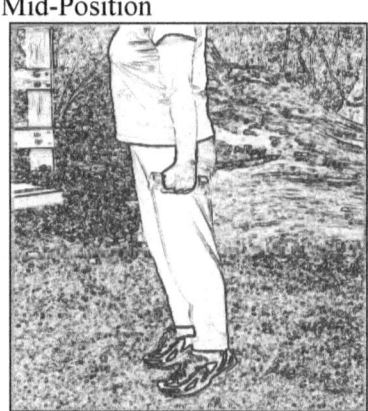

These pictures shows calf raise done with toes forward. To vary exercise,
these can also be done with toes pointed away from the center of the body or
toward the center as in pigeon toeing.

Routine Two

1-Lateral Arm Raise – one to three sets of 10 repetitions

Lateral Arm Raise

Start/End Position   Mid-Position

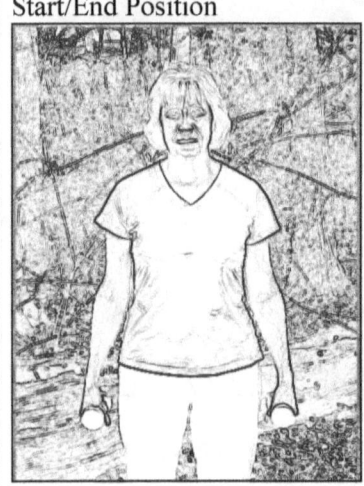
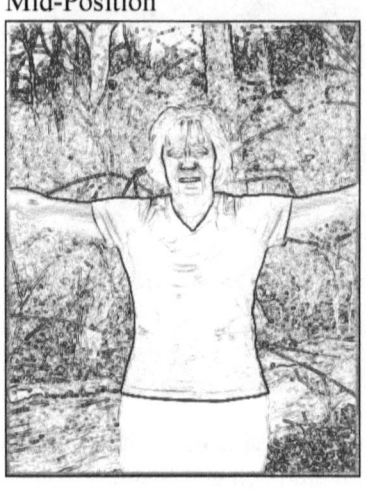

2-Bent Over Shoulder Extension With Straight Arm – one to three sets of 10 repetitions

Bent Over Shoulder Extension With Straight Arm

Start/End Position   Mid-Position

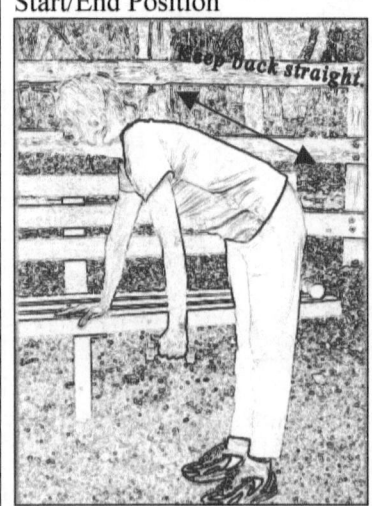
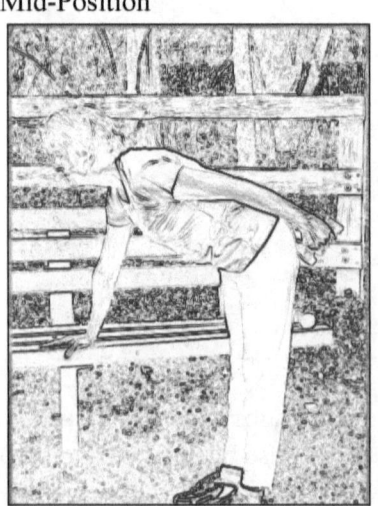

Make sure to look up during exercise; this will help keep back straight.

3-Bent Over Horizontal Abduction – one to three sets of 10 repetitions

Bent Over Horizontal Abduction

Start/End Position   Mid-Position

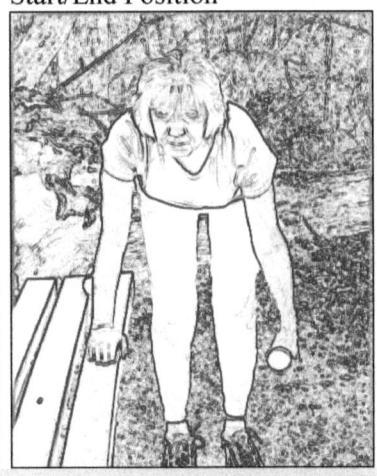 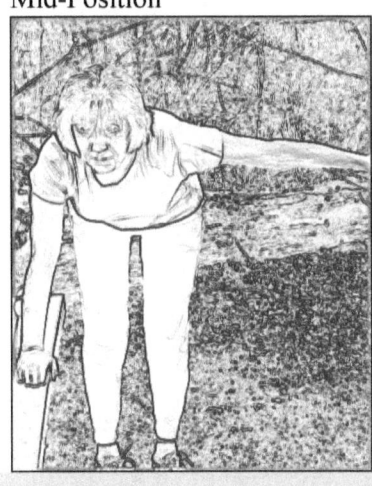

Again, remember to keep back straight.

4-Hammer Curl – one to three sets of 10 repetitions

Arm Curls With Palms Facing Each Other(Hammer Curls)

Start/End Position   Mid-Position

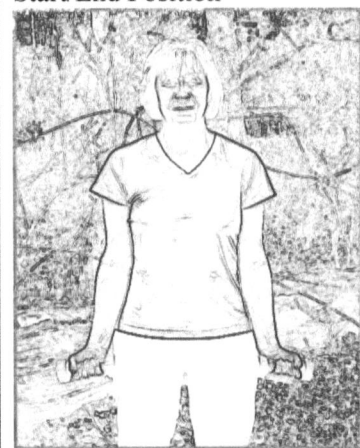 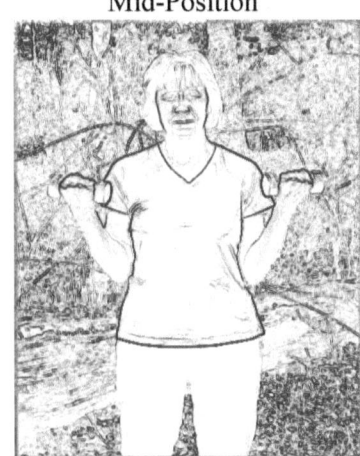

<u>Hammer Curl (Arm Curl With Palms Facing each other)</u> as shown, except with palms facing each other and thumbs up- as in swinging a hammer.

5-Pushup Pivoting Off Of Knees With Hands Wide – one to three sets of 10 repetitions

Pushup Pivoting Off Of Knees With Hands Wide

Start/End Position   Mid-Position

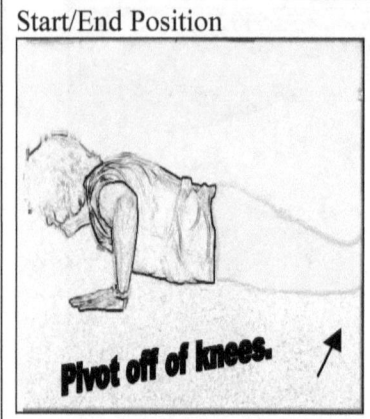 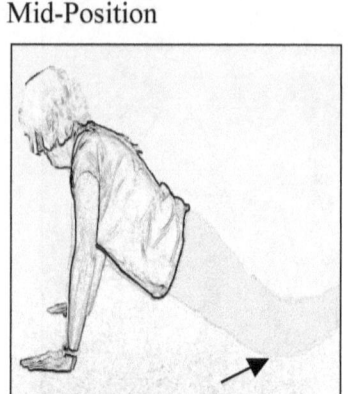

Pushup Pivoting Off Of Knees With Hands Wide is performed as above, but with hands one palm width wider than shoulders.

6- Standing Triceps Extension – one to three sets of 10 repetitions

Standing Triceps Extension

Start/End Position   Mid-Position

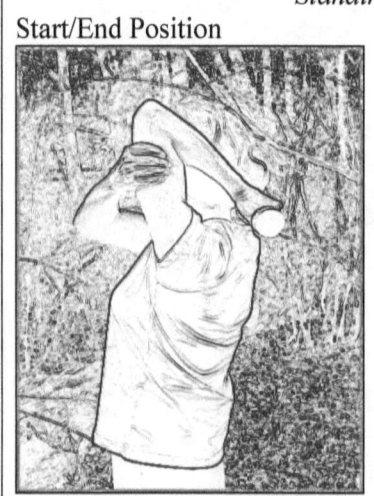 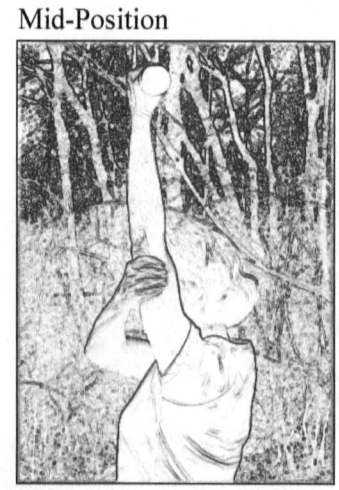

7- Abdominal Crunch With Twist – one to three sets of 10 repetitions

Abdominal Crunch With Twist

Start/End Position   Mid-Position

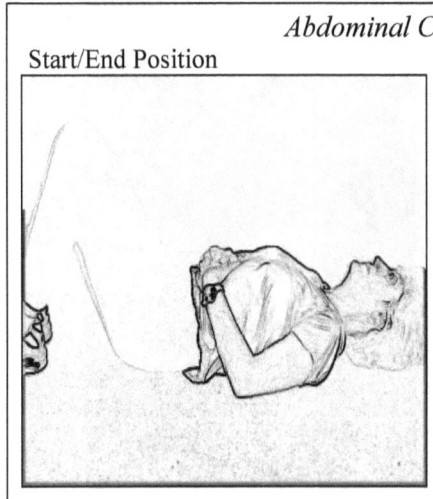 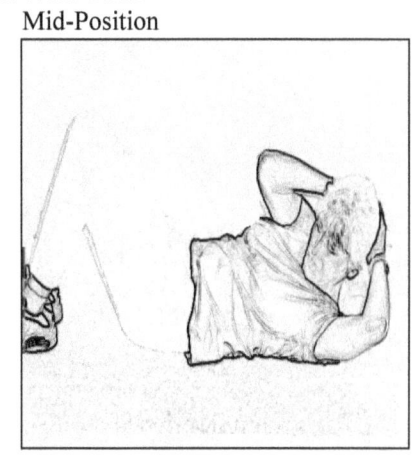

8-Quadruped Kick Back – one to three sets of 10 repetitions

Quadruped Kick Backs (on hands and knees)

Start/End Position   Mid-Position

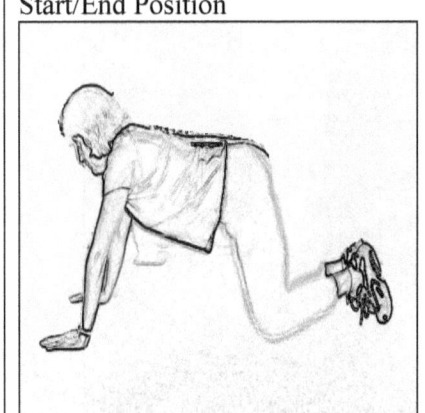 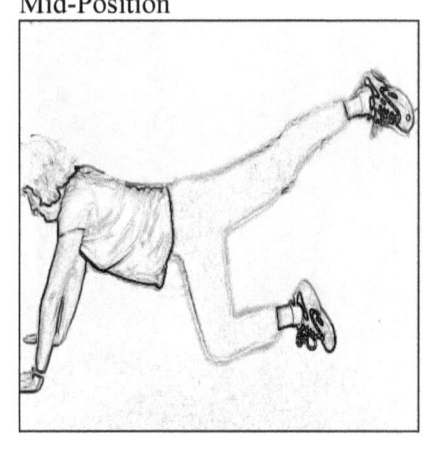

9-Lunge – one to three sets of 10 repetitions

Lunge

Start/End Position   Mid-Position

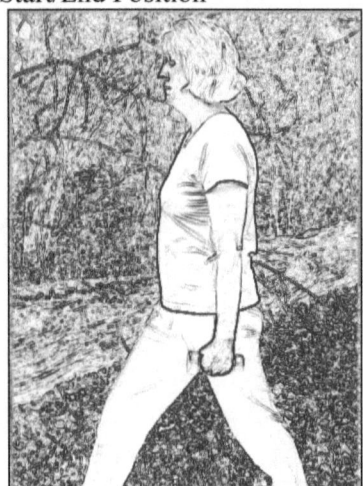
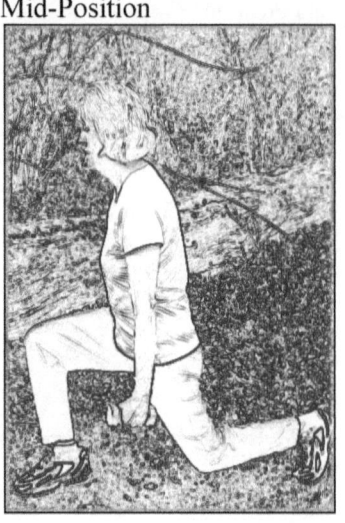

10-Standing Calf Raise (toes out) – one to three sets of 10 repetitions

Standing Calf Raise (toes pointed forward/inward/outward)

Start/End Position   Mid-Position

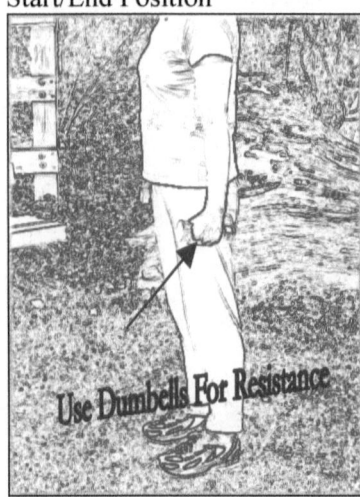
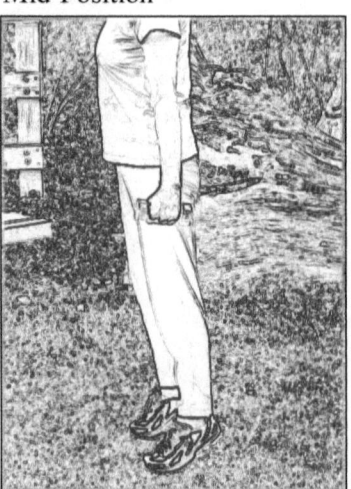

Routine Three

1-Bent Over Shrug – one to three sets of 10 repetitions

Bent Over Shrug

Start/End Position   Mid-Position

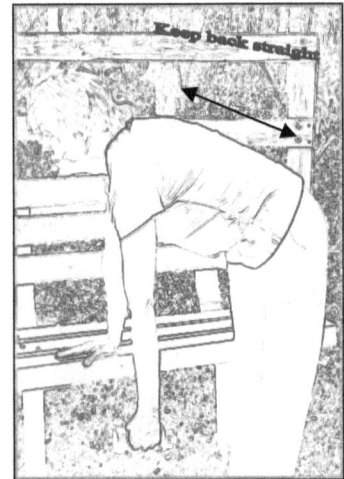 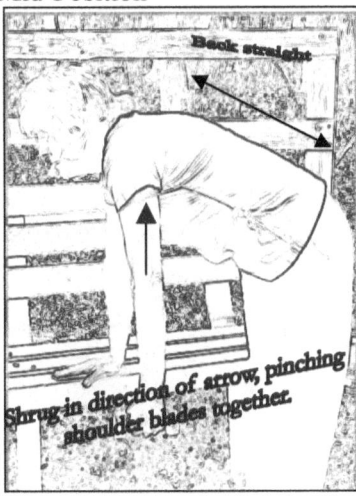

Keep elbow straight and pull arm straight up as if pinching shoulder blades together. **Be sure to keep lower back straight during this exercise**.

2-Shoulder Flexion – one to three sets of 10 repetitions

Shoulder Flexion

Start/End Position   End Position

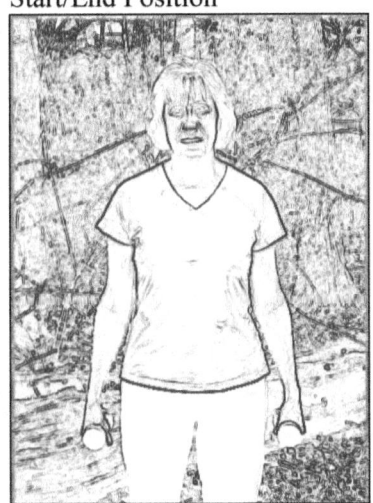 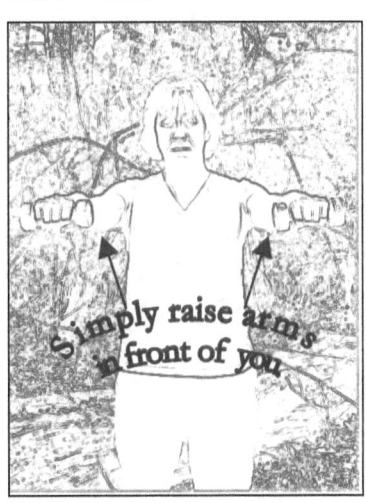

3-Standing Shoulder Extension With Bent Elbow
– one to three sets of 10 repetitions

Standing Shoulder Extension With Bent Elbow

Start/End Position   Mid-Position

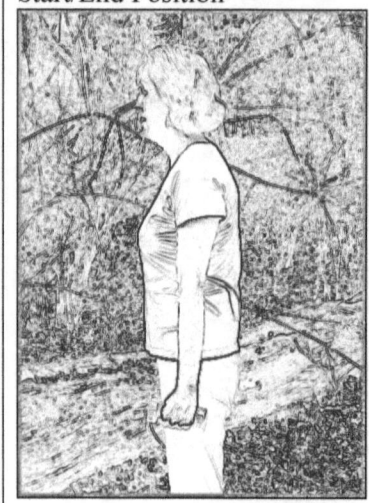 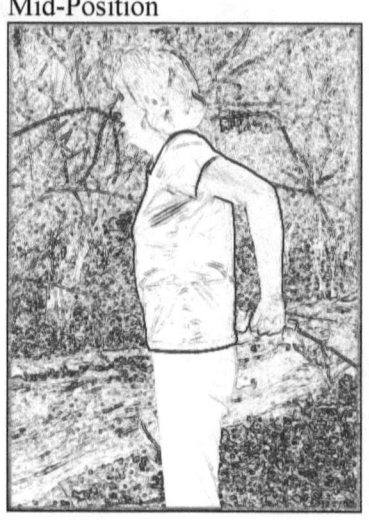

4-Seated Concentration Curl – one to three sets of 10 repetitions

Seated Concentration Curl

Start/End Position   Mid-Position

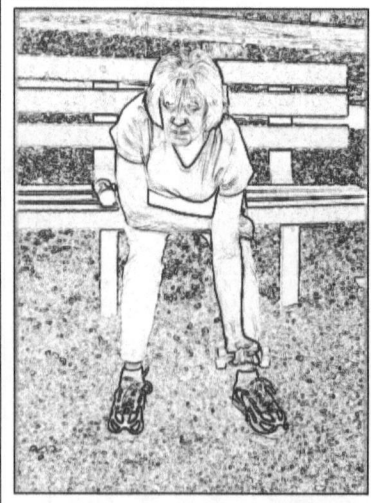 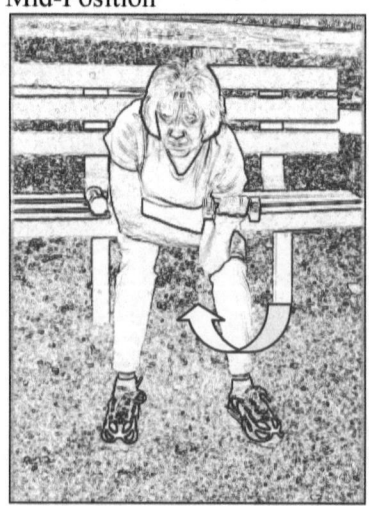

5-Arm Curl With Palms Down – one to three sets of 10 repetitions

Arm Curls With Palms Down

Start/End Position   Mid-Position

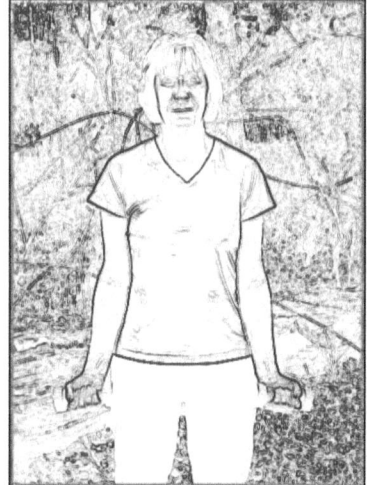 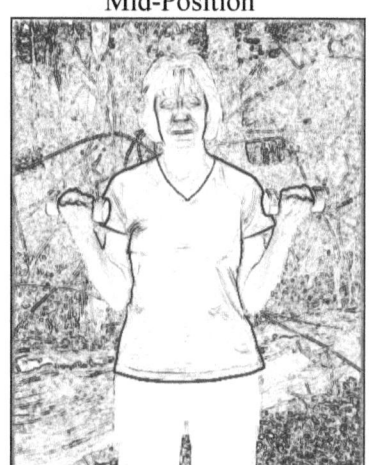

<u>Arm Curl With Palms Down</u>, *a*s per picture except with palms facing down.

6-Pushup Pivoting Off Of Knees With Knees Elevated, Hands Wide – one to three sets of 10 repetitions

Pushup Pivoting Off Of Knees With Knees Elevated, Hands One Palm Width Wider Than Shoulder Width

Start/End Position   Mid-Position

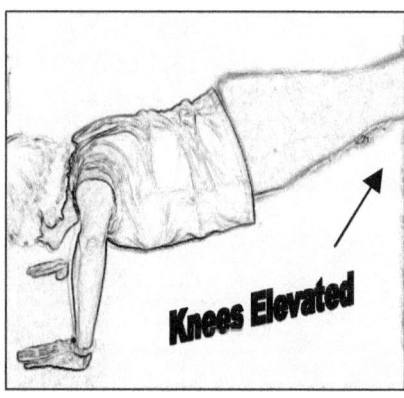 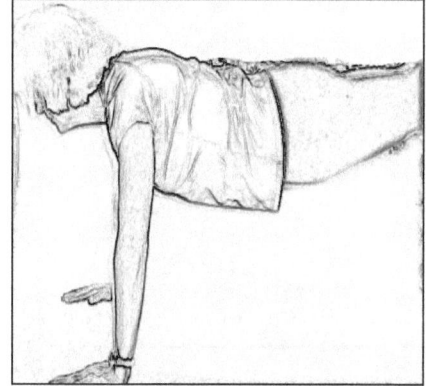

Elevate knees, as on edge of chair with cushion, and knees bent.

7-Seated Shoulder Blade Pinch – one to three sets of 10 repetitions

Seated Shoulder Blade Pinch

Start/End Position   Mid-Position

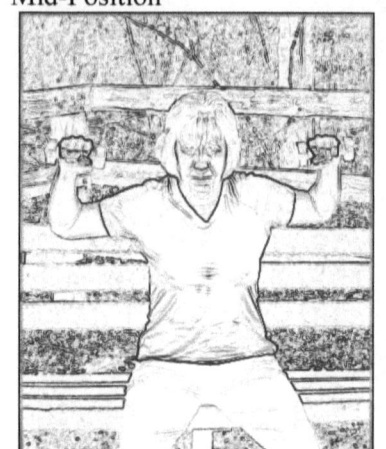

Be sure to keep chin level during this exercise.

8-Bridge With Feet Away From Body – one to three sets of 10 repetitions

Bridge with Feet Away From Body

Start/End Position   Mid-Position

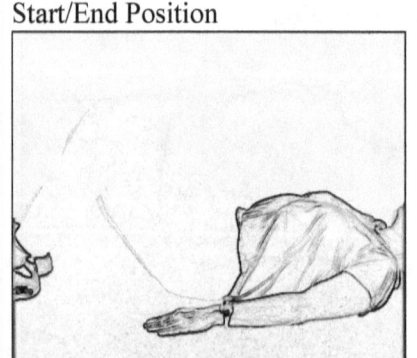
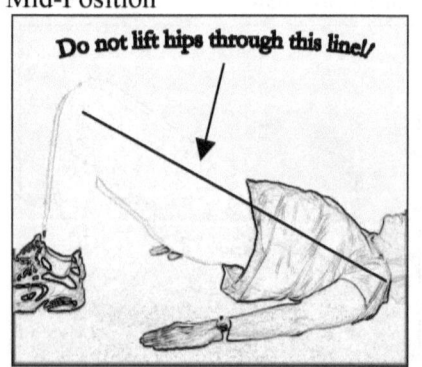

Do not lift hips through this line!

Lift hips up from the floor. Do not lift past the point where the knee, hip and shoulder form a straight line.

9-Single Leg Raise – one to three sets of 10 repetitions

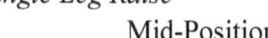

Single Leg Raise

Start/End Position   Mid-Position

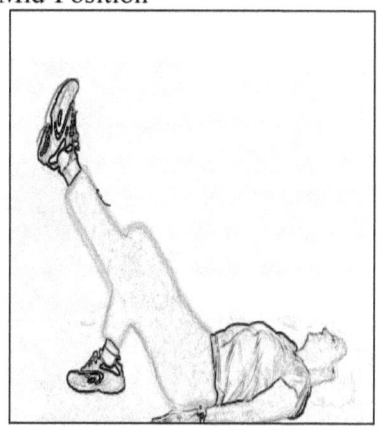

To protect your back, make sure you bend the opposite knee while doing this exercise.

10-Seated Knee Extension – one to three sets of 10 repetitions

Seated Knee Extension

Start/End Position   Mid-Position

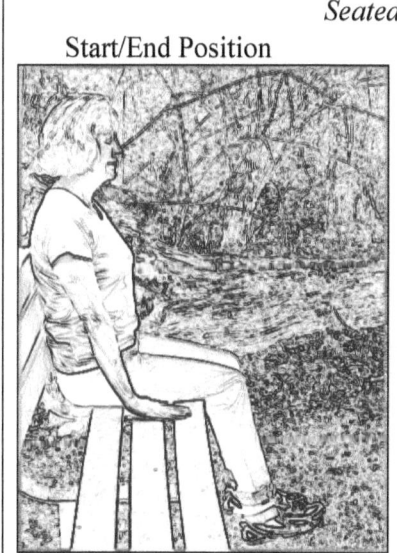
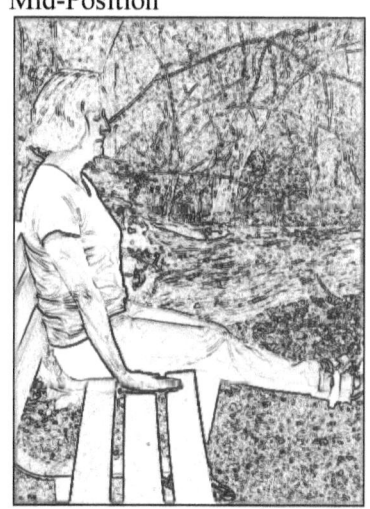

From a seated position, straighten knee.

11-Seated Calf Raise – one to three sets of 10 repetitions

Seated Calf Raise

Start/End Position   Mid-Position

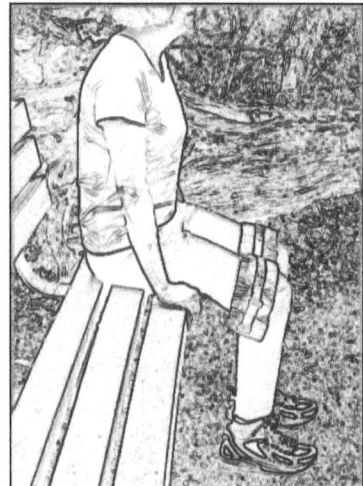 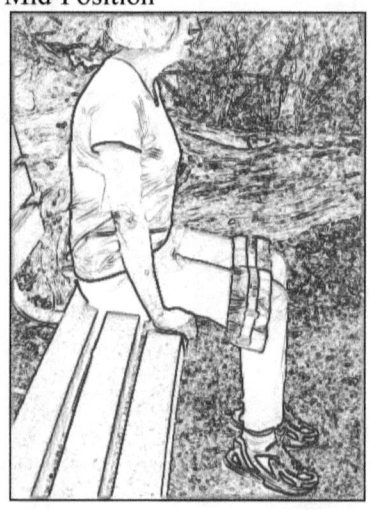

These are powerful muscles and, believe it or not, you can have a friend sit on your knees for resistance. Those are ankle weights draped across the subject's knees. To increase effectiveness, a board can be placed under the toes.

Routine Four

1-Scaption – one to three sets of 10 repetitions

Scaption

Start/End Position   Mid-Position

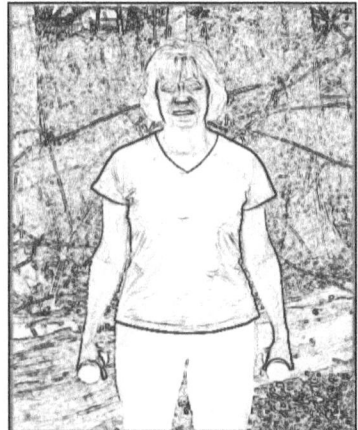 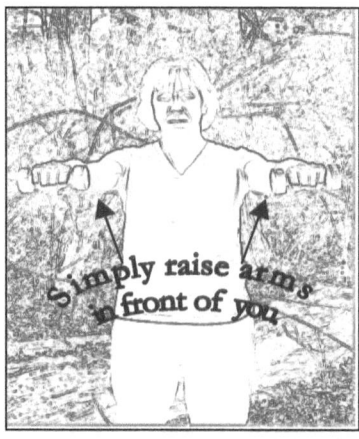

Raise arms up as in shoulder flexion, but spread arms out until they are at a 45-degree angle to your body. Think halfway between raising arms straight forward and raising them out to the side.

2-Prone Shoulder Rotation – one to three sets of 10 repetitions

Prone Shoulder Rotation

External Shoulder Rotation   Internal Shoulder Rotation

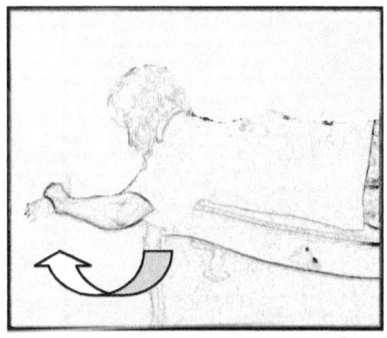 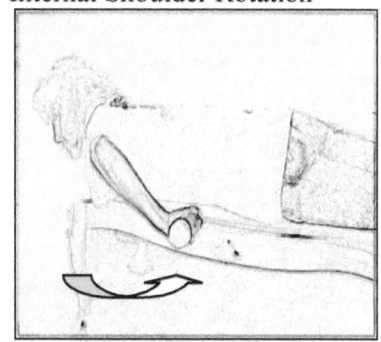

Lie on stomach with arm out to side so elbow is at edge of surface. Rotate shoulder per diagram.

3-Bent Over Shoulder Extension With Straight Arm – one to three sets of 10 repetitions

Bent Over Shoulder Extension with Straight Arm

Start/End Position	Mid-Position

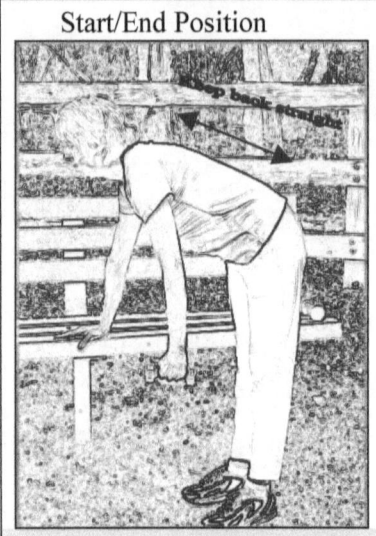 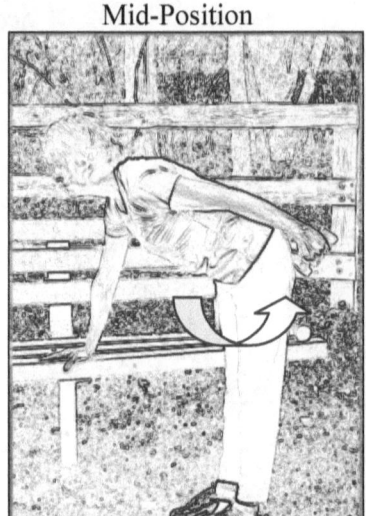

Make sure you look up while doing exercise. This will help to keep your back straight.

4-Supine Triceps Extension – one to three sets of 10 repetitions

Supine Triceps Extension

Start/End Position	Mid-Position

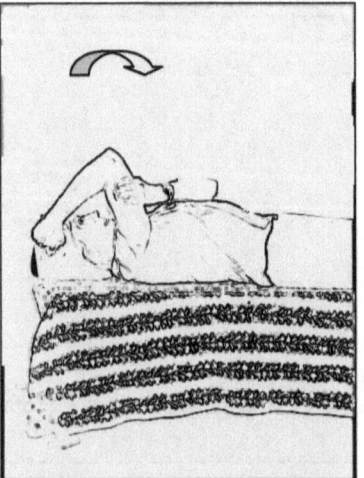 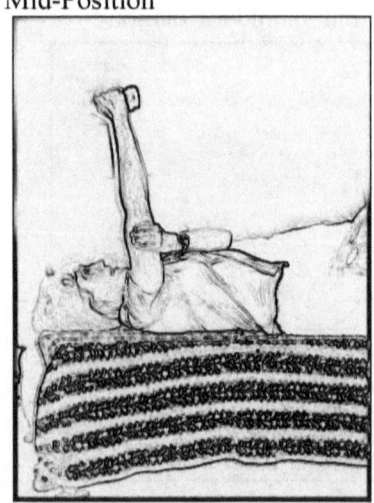

Do one arm at a time. Support with opposite hand per picture.

5-Traditional Pushup – one to three sets of 10 repetitions

Traditional Pushup

Start/End Position   Mid-Position

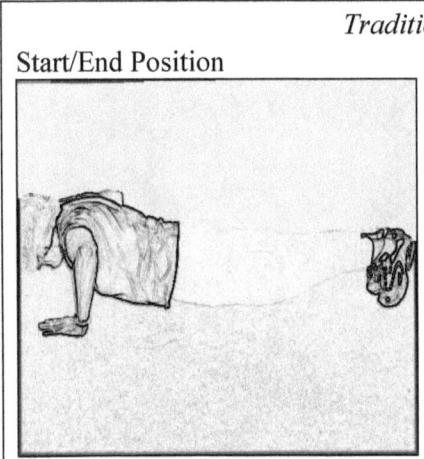
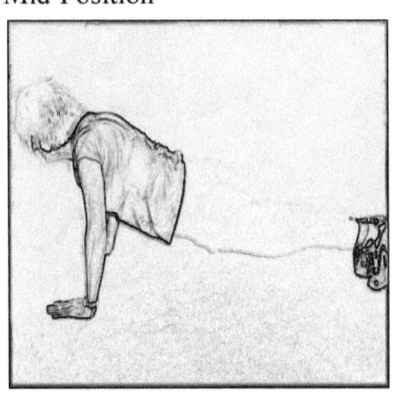

6- Elbow Curl With Shoulders Flexed – one to three sets of 10 repetitions

Elbow Curls With Shoulders Flexed

Start/End Position   Mid-Position

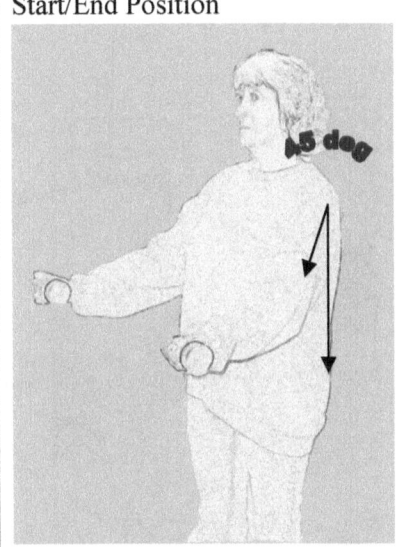
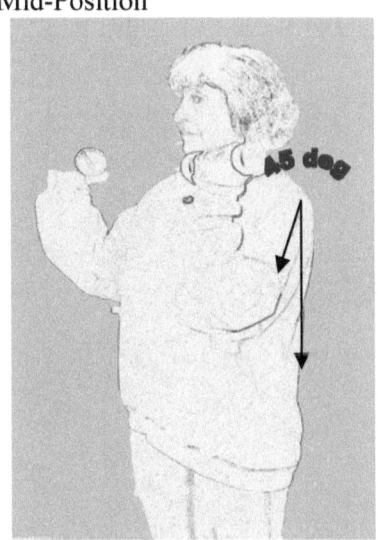

Flex shoulders forward to approximately 45 degrees, and while holding this position, curl and extend elbows. Do not allow arms to go down to your side until set is done.

7-Wrist Flexion – one to three sets of 10 repetitions

Wrist Flexion

Start/End Position   Mid-Position

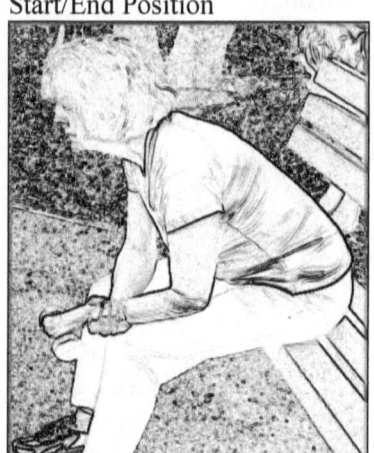 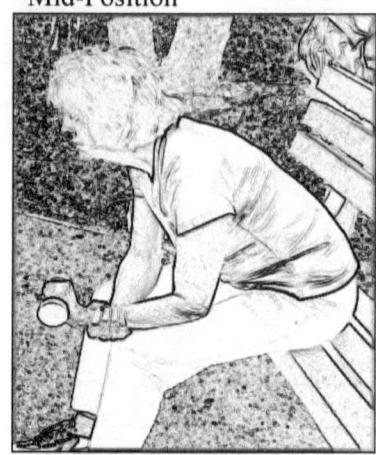

This picture illustrates wrist extension.   Notice the palm is down and supported by the opposite hand, for <u>Wrist flexion</u> the palm is up.

8-Wrist Extension – one to three sets of 10 repetitions

Wrist Extension

Start/End Position   Mid-Position

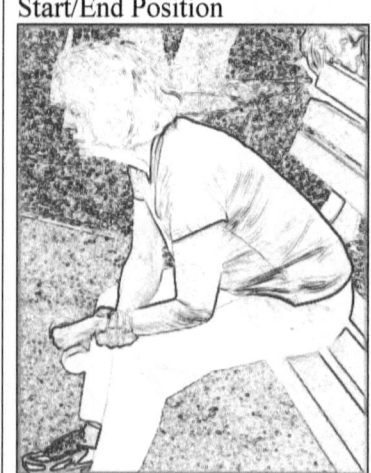 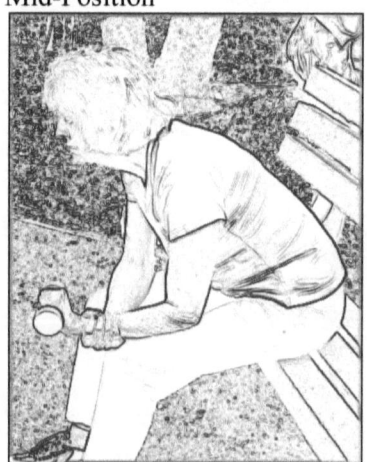

This picture illustrates wrist extension.   Notice the palm is down and supported by the opposite hand, for <u>Wrist flexion</u> the palm would be up.

9-Bridge With Feet Close – one to three sets of 10 repetitions

Bridge With Feet Close To Body

Start/End Position   Mid Position

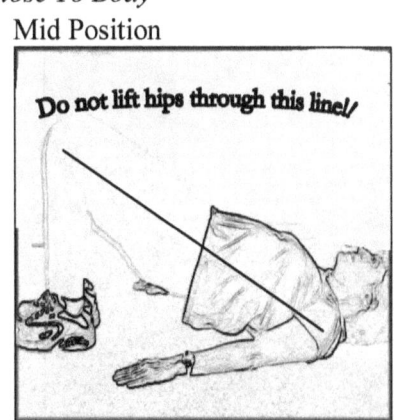

10-Single Leg Kick – one to three sets of 10 repetitions

Single Leg Kick

Start/End Position   Mid Position

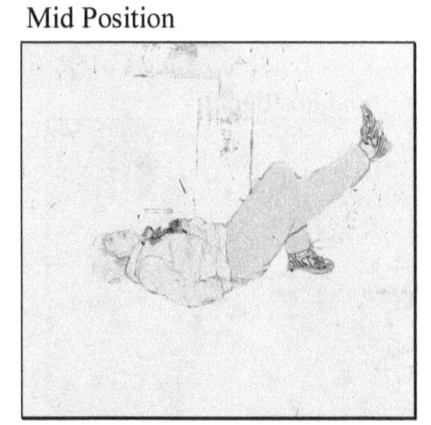

Hands should be placed under outside of buttocks to support lower back. Kick leg out until fully extended, hold for one second. **If you have any history of back injury, back pain or previous leg pain, especially extending from the back, do not do this exercise.**

11-Full Squat – one to three sets of 10 repetitions

Squat- Half/Full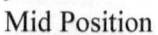

Start/End Position   Mid Position

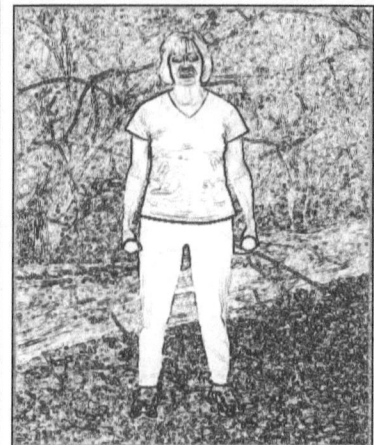 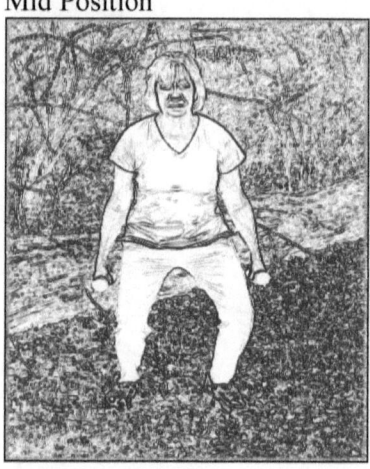

Here we illustrate the <u>half-squat</u> with knees bent to approx 45 degrees in the mid-position. To do the <u>Full squat</u> you would bend to 90 degrees in the mid-position, or about twice as far.

12-Standing Calf Raise (toes forward) – one to three sets of 10 repetitions

Standing Calf Raise (toes pointed forward)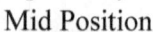

Start/End Position   Mid Position

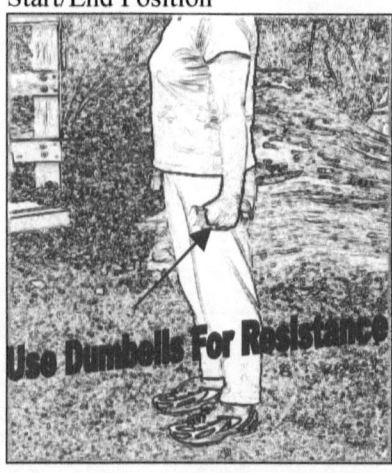 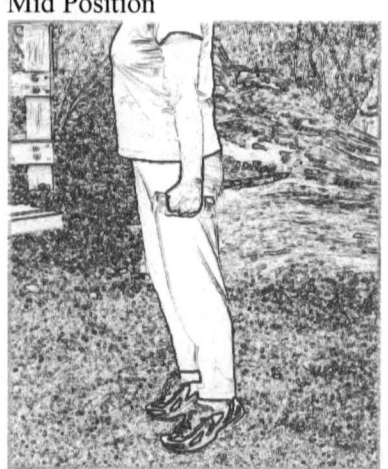

This picture shows calf raise done with toes forward.

Aerobic Exercise Examples

Aerobic Dance	Ski Machine
Bicycling	Stair Climb
Elliptical Machine	Swimming
Running	Walking

Tip: Aerobic exercise increases the number of calories your body uses for a few hours after the exercise.

The aforementioned routines can serve as good starting points. Those of you with more equipment will, of course, have more choices. The reason four sample protocols are provided is to illustrate how one might change their program four times per year, or seasonally. This is similar to the seasonal approach used with the aerobic exercises mentioned previously in this chapter. If you decide to follow these routines, you should find that, with 30-second rest periods between sets, you are able to finish the routine in 25 – 30 minutes. Remember, especially when first starting, use light weights and focus on proper execution, or form, when doing the exercise. If you have any doubts about whether or not you are doing an exercise correctly, refer back to the pictures in this chapter, and/or consult an exercise professional.

Prior to starting any exercise session, it is a good idea to warm up the muscle groups you will be exercising on that day. This could simply consist of one or two light sets before using significant resistance, i.e., if you are doing squats while holding two ten-pound dumbbells, do a set with no weights first.

Some fitness professionals also recommend stretching the individual muscles you will be working in that session. If you do stretch, be very careful not to use too much force, and always do a general warm-up before stretching. Adopting these habits can improve your flexibility and assist in the prevention of injuries.

In this chapter, I have tried to give you some of the basic knowledge necessary to start an exercise program. I have assumed that the average reader of this book will be new to exercise and have little equipment, so these recommendations are geared to that circumstance. As we discussed in the beginning of this chapter, there are many ways to approach exercise, depending on your goals, fitness level, access to equipment, and time available. This section is meant to infect the novice with one of the best addictions one can have by starting them out slowly and easily, and showing that, with persistence, amazing results can occur.

Remember, these are just sample routines; I am not recommending that you follow these specific protocols, and they do not represent the only way these exercises can be combined. There are many factors to consider when planning an exercise program, including general conditioning, pre-existing health or orthopedic problems, and fitness goals, just to name a few. If you have any doubts about setting up your own program, you should consult a fitness professional, and again, *ALWAYS CONSULT YOUR DOCTOR BEFORE BEGINNING ANY NEW EXERCISE PROGRAM*.

5 | Putting It All Together

Small Steps Can Take You Far

If you're worried about Phil and Gloria, don't be. They're doing fine and we will be taking an in-depth look at them and exactly how they have implemented this approach into their respective lifestyles before the end of this chapter. Before we do that, however, let's read through this summation of The Part-Time Diet Approach.

Believe it or not, you have come a long way in a short time. You have learned why traditional diets don't work, and how to trick your body into cooperating with your weight loss efforts. You have learned to count calories without making yourself crazy, and you have learned how to put the principles of part-time dieting to work for you. Last, but certainly not least, you have learned the basics of exercise and why it is critical to permanent weight loss. Now, you are ready to tie all the elements together into a comprehensive program, and put it to use in your daily routine. In other words, you have reached the "nuttiest and boltiest" (remember, back in the preface and again in chapter-one you were promised a nuts and bolts approach) part of the program.

To help you get started, I have condensed this plan into six simple steps outlined below. After that, we will revisit Gloria and Phil to see precisely how they incorporated this approach into their lives. Although Gloria and Phil are fictitious composites of people we have known, it is my hope that these examples will give you a preview of what to expect when you start on your own program. These examples definitely do not represent the only way to use this plan. If I have outlined this approach correctly, you will see the flexibility that is an integral part of it, and eventually learn how to apply it to your unique lifestyle. Now, let's start at the beginning.

S tep One – Determine your DCN. Use the BMR table or the formula to find your BMR and apply the correct multiplier. Since making you turn back to chapter two to find the correct multiplier would have only burned a few calories anyway, I decided to paste the table here.

-If you are Sedentary (little or no exercise)
Calorie-Calculation = BMR X 1.2
-If you are Lightly Active (light exercise/sports 1-3
days/week) Calorie-Calculation = BMR X 1.375
-If you are Moderately Active (moderate exercise/sports 3-5
days/week) Calorie-Calculation = BMR X 1.55
-If you are Very Active (hard exercise/sports 6-7
days/week) Calorie-Calculation = BMR X 1.725
-If you are Extra Active (very hard daily exercise/sports &
physical job or 2X day training) Calorie-Calculation = BMR
X 1.9

So again, if your BMR is 1686 calories per day, and you do little exercise, your DCN is 1686 X 1.2 or 2023 calories per day.

Step Two – Do you remember the four rules mentioned for weight loss way back in chapter two? This step will incorporate the first three of those rules. That is: you will subtract enough calories from any three or four days per week to create a weekly shortage of 3500. You will not diet more than four days per week, and you will eat your full DCN on the others.

As mentioned before, if you have been yo-yo dieting on a regular basis, starting this program by eating your full DCN for seven days is often a good first step. Among other benefits, this can also help determine if your DCN calculation is correct. If you start the program this way, by the third full-DCN day, you should have no chronic hunger (hunger not satisfied after meals) and after the seventh day, you should have gained no more than the pound or two that can be expected from "water weight"; often there is no weight gain at all. If you were to continue eating your DCN for longer than a week, say a month or two, there should be no more weight gain after the first week, as long as your activity level stays the same. This, again, agrees with the notion that a good way to define your DCN is: it is the number of calories that prevents hunger and does not cause weight gain.

If you are really small, creating a 3500-calorie deficit per week may be very difficult using this system. You certainly can still use this approach, but you may only be able to lose one-half to two-thirds of a pound per week. Never forget that controlled and sustainable body fat loss has a much better chance of being permanent than quick weight loss. If you are losing a half-pound per week, and virtually 100 percent of it is fat, this is better than losing a pound or more per week where as much as one-third is muscle. Keep in mind, you only want to do this once, because repeated weight loss increases body fat every time you go through the lose-weight-gain-weight cycle, and body fat uses virtually no calories compared to muscle. Studies also show this weight cycling can be devastating to your immune system, and even contribute to diabetes and some forms of heart disease in women.

Step Three – This is really an expansion of the fourth rule we discussed back in chapter two. That is: you will now decide exactly which exercises you will employ. This can be as simple as flipping back to chapter four, picking a routine and getting started. Remember, you should use a combination of aerobic exercise to promote burning of body fat, and anaerobic exercise to maintain muscle tissue. Also, try to do anaerobic (weight lifting) exercise on full-DCN days; it helps with muscle maintenance. What about those of you who can only start with a walking program? The answer to that question is an emphatic: This is fine too, where you start is insignificant, where you finish is what counts.

Step Four – Monitor your weight once per week. This must be done under the same conditions every time. We would suggest weighing yourself in the morning, after any bathroom necessities, and before you eat. This should also be done on the same day each week, on the same scale, wearing the same clothes or, better yet, no clothes. Generally, the most consistent time to weigh-in is the morning after the last light-day in a given week. For example, if you decide Monday, Tuesday and Wednesday will be your light-days then you would weigh yourself on Thursday morning before you eat or drink anything. If you split your light-days up like: Sunday, Tuesday and Thursday, then Friday morning would be the best day to weigh yourself.

Despite what you just read, in the interest of completeness, it should be mentioned that, if you're brave, you can weigh yourself every day, but be aware that your weight will fluctuate day to day. Many diets "gurus" tell you not to do this because watching your weight rise and fall can drive some people to acute caloric overload, i.e., "pig out" followed by catastrophic diet failure.

Under certain circumstances, though, we think the information you glean from this can be useful. For example, most people group the light-days together and weigh-in on the morning of the first full-day before they have eaten. This is usually the lightest you will be for that week, but let's just say you've eaten something salty, like canned soup, on the day before weigh-in. This may cause you to retain water and appear as though you have lost no weight for that week. If you then avoid excess salt and weigh yourself the next day, you may see that you have indeed lost the weight you expected. By weighing yourself every day, you will become familiar with your body's patterns and be less likely to panic if it looks like your weight loss efforts have stalled.

You may even want to keep a journal to see how certain foods affect you. For example, recently, this author had gotten into the habit of eating a take out ice cream cone two or three times a week for a few weeks, and then noticed that weight loss slowed dramatically. After taking home and weighing the offending snack, it was discovered that instead of the 350 calories at which it was guesstimated, it should have been counted as 600 calories. After relegating this to a very occasional snack, weight loss resumed at a more normal pace.

One more situation where daily weigh-ins can be useful is in helping women identify weight fluctuations caused by their menstrual cycle. Most women are aware of the bloating and temporary weight gain caused by their monthly shift in hormones, but not everyone has actually measured how much weight fluctuation it causes. Daily weigh-ins can help you determine exactly how many pounds you lose or gain, and on what days to expect this. Having this knowledge can help you calculate your true weight, and save a lot of frustration when the scale shows higher numbers than you might expect. Remember, although daily weigh-ins may be useful, it is not for the faint of heart. Do whatever suits your personality the best.

Step Five – If you find that weight loss has plateaued, modify your caloric intake and/or exercise routine. Notice, I did not say decrease calories and increase exercise. It is much more effective to change a program than to just add exercises or eat less.

Step Six – If your weight refuses to budge, no matter what calorie deficit pattern you throw at it, simply eat your full DCN for one week and then resume some combination of light and full-days the following week. I like to call this the "vacation clause" as it, in effect, allows you to take a vacation from your weight loss efforts. You can also use this clause if you really are going on vacation and do not want to diet during that time; just don't eat more than your DCN.

Some Intimate Facts About Gloria?

B y now, you probably feel that you know Gloria pretty well, but for the purposes of this section, you will need to learn more about some of her physical attributes. Essentially, she was cobbled together from experiences and comments that have been related to us from people who have tried this approach. Gloria is a typical female who wants to lose weight, but who is also starting to resign herself to the fact that she may never be able to achieve this goal. As you've probably guessed, she is a little past 40-years old, and over the last ten years, she has watched her once-svelte figure sag and stretch from age and childbearing.

Gloria has tried basically every diet there is with only temporary success. One time, she was actually able to attain her target weight, but the minute she tried to resume a more normal eating regimen, she was slowly pulled by the demons of genetics and a lowered BMR back up to her previous weight, plus ten pounds. She has also tried exercise, but it was mostly geared to aerobic and it actually contributed to muscle loss. During these cycles, though, she did manage to achieve one semipermanent change in her body. Every time she came full circle and reached her old weight, she had achieved a higher percentage of body fat.

As you might recall, at the outset of this approach, Gloria was skeptical and leery of yet another diet plan that might result in more failure. This is why we (Danielle) had to lure her in to our way of thinking by just having her cut her calories in half a few days per week. This proved to her that dieting need not be done every day to be effective.

When Gloria started this system, she stood five feet four inches in height, and weighed 160 pounds. She had a sedentary job and all the demands of family life.   After looking up her BMR (for the sake of continuity of the story, let's again say Danielle) found Gloria should burn 1457 calories per day at rest. After multiplying by 1.2, she calculated that, under Gloria's then activity level, she needed 1748 calories per day to maintain her body weight. Or, rounding up, we can say her DCN back then was 1750 calories per day. Incidentally, her initial reaction was that she already ate less than that and wasn't losing any weight. Attentive readers now know what would have been the correct response to her protestation: Gloria, your metabolism needs a good swift kick!

Gloria's initial exercise program consisted of riding a stationary bike for one-half hour per day, three days per week, and performing a one-half hour anaerobic exercise program three days per week. Because she was still in rehab, she had access to a pretty comprehensive set of machines and equipment, so changing the routine was no problem. Now that rehab is over, and she has little in the way of equipment at home, she has chosen to follow the first routine mentioned in chapter four, twice per week. You remember, right? OK, I'll save you the lookup time:

Shoulder Shrugs – one to three sets of 10 repetitions
Shoulder Press – one to three sets of 10 repetitions
Arm Curls Palms Up – one to three sets of 10 repetitions
Arm Curls Palms Down – one to three sets of 10 repetitions
Pushups Pivoting Off of Knees with Hands Shoulder Width – one to three
                                 sets of 10 repetitions
One Arm Dumbbell Row – one to three sets of 10 repetitions
Squat/Clean – one to three sets of 10 repetitions
Abdominal Crunches – one to three sets of 10 repetitions
Half-Squats – one to three sets of 10 repetitions
Standing Leg Curls – one to three sets of 10 repetitions (ankle weights or
                              heavy shoes can be used for resistance)
Standing Calf Raise – one to three sets of 10 repetitions

The aerobic portion of her exercise simply consisted of walking for one-half hour per day, five days per week. Since she remained true to this program, her DCN had actually gotten a bit higher than previously quoted. In fact, her multiplier was now a conservative 1.37, which yields a DCN of a little over 1996 calories per day. When we told "Gloria" this, we could see the twinkle in her eyes, as she suppressed a smile. Feeling this was too good to be true though, she decided to stay in the 1900 calorie per day range. She did not have time for any other exercise then, so she had to work within these parameters.

With regard to her eating program, Gloria had decided she would use four light-days and three full-days for her caloric approach. She found that Sunday through Wednesday worked best for her light-days. This meant Thursday, Friday, and Saturday would be her full DCN days. Gloria could have chosen any four days of the week for her light-days, but these just happened to suit her schedule the best. If she had decided to use Sunday, Tuesday, Wednesday and Thursday, the program would work just as well.

Gloria chose to eat 1000 calories on her light-days and 1900 calories on her full-days. This produced a weekly shortage of 3600 calories, using her self-imposed 1900-calorie limit on full days. In reality, the deficit was closer to 4300, since her true caloric need was closer to 2000. On her light days she was really eating 1000 calories less than she needed, and on her full days she was still 100 calories light. If you add up the deficits, you would see that since she removed 1000 on four light days, plus 100 calories per day on each of her three full days, she actually ended up with a 4300-calorie shortage.

Following this plan caused her to lose an average of slightly more than one pound per week. At the risk of sounding pedantic, I will reiterate: this program focuses on <u>sustainable</u> loss of body fat while preserving muscle, so rate of weight loss is secondary to quality of weight loss.

Armed with these numbers, Gloria was then ready to begin what she hoped would be her last weight reduction program. She was a bit nervous, and part of her wanted to retreat to her old habits of skipping breakfast, salad for lunch and chicken breast for dinner, but she didn't because she knew this always eventually failed. Now, let's zoom in on Gloria and see how she might have actually handled those first months of her new lifestyle.

It is Sunday morning, the first day of her new plan, and her kitchen is redolent of a home-cooked breakfast. The individual aromas of scrambled eggs, toast, and coffee harmonize to play a symphony for the olfactory sense. Gloria knows she won't have time to do this every day, but she thought, just for today, she would get up a little early and start this new approach on a positive note. The kids seem to approve as they stumble into the kitchen, first her six-year-old daughter Jennifer, and then her eight-year-old son Ryan, both with the same quizzical smiles on their faces.

"Mom, if this is your new diet, I can't wait until I need to lose weight," says Ryan.

For this morning's breakfast, Gloria decides to have one scrambled egg, a piece of whole grain toast with a light butter substitute that her doctor has told her actually reduces cholesterol, and six ounces of orange juice. She has already taken the two minutes necessary to research this, and she knows that the total calories in this meal are approximately 310. She is off to an excellent start.

After breakfast, Gloria busies herself with her daily operations. Her mother-in-law has taken the kids to their various activities, and by-and-by, she finds herself alone in the house. Over the sounds of vacuuming, dusting and straightening, she involuntarily begins to tune into it, "it" being a subtle undercurrent that carries an old and familiar song, a song she feels quite sure is being sung by the many cookies, cupcakes and boxes of holiday candy stored in the various cupboards around the house. "We are your fun time, your only fun time, we make you happy, when you are blue." Gloria smiles and turns on the stereo in the living room, thinking, *'Just a few days, my friends, in just a few days, I can eat you if I really want to.'* Knowing that she could theoretically fit "junk food" into her program buoys her even though the old dieter in her advises against it, at least in the beginning. A half-hour before lunch, she decides to take her walk. Although it is early January, the temperature is in the low forties and the sun is shining. Walking is something she has been focusing on since her knee surgery, so she is able to do a full half-hour. Thanks to her headphones, the time passes quickly and she feels refreshed when she returns. After shaking off the cold, she prepares lunch, which consists of a bowl of chicken soup and half of a ham and cheese sandwich with wholegrain bread, one slice of cheese, one ounce of ham and light mayonnaise. Total calorie count for this meal is 300. For her drink, she decides to just have water with this meal. She could have had any diet drink, or coffee, or tea, or even half of a glass of skim milk, but choosing water allows her to save a few extra calories for supper.

An hour later, Gloria's mother-in-law and kids return home. They eat the same foods she did, albeit in less precise amounts, and then settle into their various routines, i.e. kids to homework and Judy to her weekly crossword puzzle. Presently, Judy decides to make hot cocoa for the kids. Since she doesn't want to "spend" her calories on this, Gloria decides to walk to her sister Josephine's house. There she has coffee and discusses her new weight loss plan.

Josephine, who has never had a weight problem, doesn't recognize that she follows the same eating pattern without thinking, and ironically, she is critical of Gloria's new strategy. After a little more brow beating, Gloria furtively rolls her eyes and looks at the clock. It is now 5:30, so Gloria phones her mother-in-law and asks her to put a casserole, she had previously prepared, into the oven. She finally leaves her sister's house feeling a little dejected. Way to go, Jo. Not!

When she arrives home, Gloria is glad that Judy has the casserole just about heated. She is hungry, and she knows if she allows herself to become too hungry, it makes it harder to stick to the plan.

Gloria had made the tuna casserole from a recipe she downloaded from the Internet. It provides 250 calories per one-cup serving. Along with it, she has steamed mixed vegetables with a little butter, and a salad with low calorie dressing. The salad and the vegetables with butter add up to a little less than 100 calories. For dessert, she has grapes. Total caloric value for this meal is just shy of 400. This gives her a total of 1000 for the day, right on the money. Again, no special preparation is necessary for her light-day. Again, her family eats what she eats, albeit a little more.

The rest of her light-days pass pretty much like this one. Gloria tries, especially on the light days, to eat different foods each day so she doesn't become bored with the meals. On Thursday morning, Gloria weighs herself and finds that she has lost two and one-half pounds. She is ecstatic, and despite her admonishing conscience, she silences the singing cookie choir in her pantry by eating two of them. No biggie, she just adds the unfortunate gingersnaps to her tally.

Another week flies by and she loses another one and a quarter pounds. This is more than she dared ask for, and even though she knows the weight loss will not always proceed at this pace, she still finds it exciting. Sure enough, after three weeks, her weight loss slows to just about a pound per week.

During this time, Gloria has noticed that although she is hungry during the light-days, it is manageable because she knows that respite is always only a few days away. She also discovers that each week after the first or second full DCN day, her hunger pangs are completely satisfied, and very often by the third full-day, she is tempted to eat less than her DCN because she is simply not hungry. She does not succumb to this temptation, though, because she knows she needs these calories to rev up her metabolism for the next cycle of light-days. I should also point out that over the last few weeks, she has gained a little more faith in the system and is now eating 2000 calories on her full DCN days, and she has increased her light days to 1100 to produce a 3600-calorie per week deficit.

Each week, Gloria's third full DCN day happens to land on Saturday, and it is on one of these Saturday afternoons that she realizes that for much of the week, she is truly not hungry, and yet she is losing weight. She smiles as it occurs to her that every Thursday represents the end of a mini-diet. A little more reverie, and her subconscious mind meanders into a wall metaphor where she sees that:

> like a wall that is constructed one brick at a time, this approach breaks the big job of losing weight into many small pieces. This, ladies and gentlemen, is the very essence of this approach!!!

Gloria continues to diet and experience consistent weight loss for approximately three months, and then she hits the bane of all diets: the plateau. Her heart sinks a little when she stands on the scale that has been her best friend for the last 12 weeks, and sees she weighs the same as last week. After stepping down, she examines her behavior for the last week and concludes that she has followed the diet to the letter. Then, when her weight doesn't budge for a second week, she knows the moment of truth is at hand.

Even though she knew from the start that this day would come, she still feels a little apprehensive. She remembers all too well how plateaus had been the beginning of the end for every other diet she had tried, and she is not convinced that she can handle this one. Fortunately, though, with the Part-Time Diet Approach, there is a step-by-step procedure to handle this. It just requires her to have the courage to change the program that has gotten her this far.

With this approach, there are a number of ways she can handle this. She could change her exercise program, notice I did not say increase it, and/or she could change her light-day calorie schedule. What this might mean is that instead of eating 1100 calories for four days, she could eat 1000 calories for two days and 1250 calories for two days to produce the 3500-calorie deficit necessary to lose a pound per week. Another possibility might be to eat 1000 calories per day for three days and 1500 calories on the fourth light-day to, again, produce the same weekly deficit. She would continue to eat her full DCN on the other days. As long as she ends up with a reasonable caloric deficit at the end of the week, almost any combination of light and full-days will work.

Interestingly, Gloria chooses to use three 900-calorie days instead of her previous four 1100-calorie days. If you do the math, you will see that this should produce a 3300-calorie per week deficit or just shy of a pound per week weight loss. Although this will produce a slightly slower rate of weight loss, it will allow her to do it by dieting only three days per week. To Gloria, this seems a little too good to be true, and after making this decision, she is a little conflicted. At once, the thought of four full DCN days both delights her, and scares her as she is not quite sure that this will not backfire and cause some weight re-gain.

To stack the deck in her favor, she also makes a change in her exercise program by switching from walking to using a stationary bike she had just been given by her sister's husband. The following week, her electronic scale still reads the same weight, but the next lower number is now flickering on the display screen. A week after that, the new lower number shines brightly and steadily on the screen. Gloria smiles broadly as she allows herself to entertain the notion of shopping for new clothes, and realizes she has now discovered that she can handle plateaus and, better yet, do it without increasing self-deprivation or martyrdom.

For Gloria, and most people, the plateau will occur. Now, if properly handled, it is just a bump in the road and something from which to learn. When she sees the resumption of weight loss from just a few changes, she realizes that she now has the tools to defeat this foe of all dieters. Instead of enduring the emotional frustration of plateauing, Gloria will just recognize what is going on and unemotionally make the changes she needs to further her weight loss.

Finally, when she is just a few pounds from her goal, Gloria finds that no matter what changes she makes, her weight barely budges. Previously, her emotions would have run the gamut from frustration to anger to dismay, and finally to resignation. From here, it would be just a short ride back up the weight-gain express elevator. This time, though, she experiences no such thing because she knows she has one more card to play. She simply eats her full DCN for a week, in a sense taking a week off from her diet, and resets her metabolic thermostat.

At the end of her "vacation" week, the scale says she has gained one pound. Even though she knew to expect this, and the weight gain is probably from fluid retention caused by the replenishment of glycogen, she is still a little concerned. The following week, she resumes her original four-light-day and three-full-day schedule; subsequently, on weigh-in, she finds that she has lost that pound plus one more. In other words, her weight loss has resumed, and she breathes a sigh of relief. Four weeks later, Gloria finally reaches her goal. She is ecstatic, but a little miffed because, by her calculations, she should have made the goal in three weeks. Here's a hint: she made a simple mistake that may indeed have hurt her ego, but did not really hurt her efforts.

Nevertheless, Gloria then began the most important part of the diet: the maintenance phase! We will revisit her in the next chapter to see why she missed her deadline, and what she discovers about herself and this approach.

Who Is Phil, Calorically?

Before we do that, though, let's take a look at our old buddy, Phil. As in Gloria's case, we need to know some of Phil's particulars to fully appreciate how this weight loss approach can be expected to work for members of the less fair gender.

As you probably surmised, Phil is a pretty husky guy who, like Gloria, has also been down the long boring road of the perpetual diet many times over his 43 years. He stands right around six feet four inches tall, and his initial weight was better than 290 pounds. Phil is also not particularly muscular, and a glance at his "pre-Part-Time" profile would have revealed that he was carrying baggage under his chin that would barely make carry-on status on any major airline.

Back then, Phil used food to mitigate the loneliness of a solitary lifestyle, and his high-stress, sedentary job, often eating big lunches and frequent snacks because on some elemental level, they made him feel loved and secure. The attentive reader, of course, knows this is false security as the very caloric excesses that make him feel good may be the same ones that bring along the side effects of diabetes, heart disease, gout, arthritis or worse.

Phil had started many diets before meeting Gloria, only to alternately triumph mightily and then fail miserably. Each time, by following the accepted dogma of just eat "right," or just give up fried food, or just skip lunch, the only changes he had managed to accomplish, like Gloria, were to increase his percent of body fat and lose muscle tissue. After opening his mind to what Gloria was trying to tell him, he realized that what she was describing was an approach to weight-loss that would, if nothing else, provide him with scheduled respite from caloric deprivation along the way. The logic could be summed up in one phrase: eat less than you need on some days and don't over eat on the others. The other benefits of maintained BMR and muscle tissue were great, if they worked, but it was the part-time nature of the program that finally convinced him to give it an honest try.

Phil's goal weight was 220 pounds. Since he had so much body weight to lose, instead of using his 290-pound starting weight to calculate his BMR, as stated in chapter two, he decided to use a number half way between his start weight and his goal weight. Using this weight – 255 pounds – his BMR turned out to be 2280 calories per day. Because he was the epitome of sedentary, he multiplied this by 1.2 to come up with his DCN, which calculated to right around 2700 calories per day.

Remember, this number is just a starting point, generated by a one-size-fits-all formula. Although it produces a fairly accurate BMR, you will almost certainly need to do some tweaking before it is absolutely correct for you. If weight-loss exceeds one pound per week for more than three weeks, and if you find you still feel between-meals hunger after the last day of your full-days cycle, then you can increase the DCN by 100 calories per full-day until weight-loss stabilizes to one pound per week.

All light and full-day calorie values will also be adjusted accordingly. For example, if you thought your DCN was 2500 calories per day and you started to lose a consistent 1.5 pounds per week, you might want to raise your DCN to 2600 calories per day and see how your body responds to the new caloric input. The changes in your heavy and light days might be something like: eat 2600 calories four days per week, and 1300 calories on the light days. Remember: to lose a pound per week, any combo will work as long as you remove 3500 calories per week on the light days, and never overeat (overeating in this example would mean eating more than 2600 calories) on the full-days.

Phil decided to cut his calories by 1000 for three days per week and 500 on a fourth day. This meant he would be eating 1700 calories on three light-days, and 2200 calories on a fourth light-day. This produced a 3500-calorie shortage over a week's time.

The math looks like this: Phil needs 2700 calories, but on his light-days only eats 1700 calories, which produces a 1000-calorie deficit per day over three light-days. On the final light-day, he eats 2200 calories to produce a 500-calorie deficit on the fourth light-day. He would eat his full 2700 the other three days. Initially, Phil refused to commit to any exercise program until he saw results from this approach. Like I said before, this can work in the beginning, but for long-term success, some form of aerobic and anaerobic exercise works best.

Fortunately, Phil is a bit obsessive, and was very precise in his calorie counting. This precision, despite the refusal to exercise, led to a pleasant surprise in the form of a three-pound weight loss after the first week. After two weeks, Phil had lost five pounds by simply following the "Part-Time Dieting Approach", and was quite happy with the result. In fact, so happy that, rather than motivating him to exercise, this caused Phil to become even more resolute in his avowed "couch potatoism".

Phil felt that if he could lose weight this effectively without sweating, why bother. If it weren't for Gloria and her feminine wiles, we are not sure if Phil would have ever done any motion that wasn't absolutely necessary for preservation of life, job or decorum. With her gentle coaxing, though, he decided he could fit a half-hour walk into his evenings, and soon discovered that this is a great way to decompress after a long, stressful day at work. Gloria's efforts probably saved the program for him, because long-term weight loss would have been hard to come by without at least some activity.

After ten weeks on the program, Phil had lost 14 pounds and was feeling great, not just because of the weight loss, but also because of how easy the full DCN days had been to follow. He also found that by incorporating the walking program, he was able to increase the number of full-days to four, and the calories consumed on these days to 3100. The reason for this was that since he was walking, he could now multiply his BMR by the second multiplier, which is 1.37. So, 1.37 times 2280 equals roughly 3100. Phil then cut his light days to three, and calories consumed on those days rose to 1900, so the calculation changed to: 3100 minus 1900 equals a 1200-calorie-per-day shortage. This allowed Phil to create a 3600-calorie weekly deficit in only three days, which was perfect for a one-pound per week weight loss.

Another ten weeks went by, and Phil, like Gloria, noticed that for the first time since he started, he had gone a week without losing any weight. He was moderately concerned by this, but with Gloria's tutelage, he knew to stick to the current program and give it another week. The following week, though, when he saw the same stubborn number pop up on the scale, Phil knew what he had to do. Keep in mind that, previously, this situation would have frustrated Phil, and it would have only been a matter of time before he would have backed up the old minivan to the nearest pizza shop and loaded up for a feeding frenzy. Not this time though, because Phil was starting to believe in this approach, and thought maybe, just maybe, he had the tools to fix this problem.

Instead of juggling his calories, like Gloria, Phil decided to take advantage of the "vacation clause" and take a week off from dieting.

Remember our definition of dieting is eating less than your DCN, so during this week, Phil ate his full DCN every day. Frankly, at the beginning of his "vacation week", Phil was not at all convinced that this tactic would work for him, but since he has already lost 24 pounds, he felt he could take a little chance. He was also a little weary after 20 weeks of dieting, so he appreciated the break.

The following week at his weigh-in, Phil saw that he had indeed gained a pound. Nervous, he resumed the three 1900-calorie-per-day and four 3100-calorie-per-day approach. On the morning of his second light-day, he was cautiously optimistic, as he had lost the pound he thought he had gained. On the morning after his third light-day, he is ecstatic since he is now a pound lighter and right on schedule.

> We Are Giving You The Worst Possible Scenario Here. If You Are Careful, And Do Not Exceed Your DCN, You May Experience No Weight Gain At All During The Vacation Week.

Remember, for Phil to have really gained a pound, he would have had to eat an extra 3500 calories over the course of the week. Since Phil adhered to the principle of eating his full DCN and no more, he could only have gained weight via water retention as a result of glycogen replenishment subsequent to eating more calories. This fact also explains why he was able to re-lose this weight so quickly.

A few months later, Phil ran into yet another plateau. This time, he decided to go back to a four light-day per week routine. On two of the days, he would eat 1900 calories, and on the other two, he would consume 2500 calories.

Let's see how this works: 3100 minus 1900 equals a 1200 calorie deficiency on two of the light-days, and 3100 minus 2500 equals a 600 calorie deficit on each of the other two light-days. If you add up the light-days, you see Phil is still cutting 3600 calories from his weekly intake, but it's spread over four days instead of three. His full DCN days remain at 3100.

For the exercise part of the program, Phil will be switching to a ski machine he found in the local newspaper's classified section. After a week on this schedule, Phil is delighted to see that his weight loss has resumed, and he likes his new arrangement because he can now juggle calories to allow the occasional dinner out with Gloria, even on a light-day, and still lose weight.

Four more months passed, and Phil was now only ten pounds from his goal. He decided, much to Gloria's chagrin, that since it is just early December, he would push this method to the limit. You see, Phil was pretty happy with the way he looked compared to, say, six months ago, and since he knows he has plenty of time to make his goal before Summer, he decides he will only diet one day per week for a while. His calorie intake for the low day will be 1500. This gave him a 1600-calorie deficit for the day, and since he was only dieting one day each week, his weekly deficit was, of course, the same 1600 calories.

In addition to the walking or skiing he had been doing, Phil also decided to use the company gym for one-half hour twice per week, so this new program should produce a roughly one-half pound per week weight loss. Again, he was a little nervous, but at the end of the month, when he saw that he had lost just shy of two pounds with very little discomfort, he was delighted.

Delighted, especially, because the weight-loss was so effortless that he didn't care if it took a little longer than the typical crash diet he used to employ. The desperation to finish the diet just wasn't there. He also realized that if you took into account the failures and retracements of the other diets, this diet actually produced quicker weight-loss over the long haul, and, best of all, he just liked the way he looked better this time. Fit and trim, instead of just smaller.

One evening in his home office, Phil was scanning budget proposals and personnel reviews. Because the work was so mind numbing, Phil found his focus shifting from the onerous tasks at hand to other more pleasant thoughts. It was during one of these dalliances that he found himself, almost involuntarily, leaning back in his chair and savoring what he had accomplished over the last few months. A wry smile tugged at his now leaner features as he realized, he had at last, managed to lose a significant amount of weight in a relatively painless fashion, and he had defeated the dreaded plateau not once, but twice.

Gloria, who was busy doing homework on the kitchen table, happened to look in on him and asked, "Penny for your thoughts?"

Gazing in her direction, still deep in thought, he said, "You know, people at work have really taken notice, and some are even grousing that I'm probably taking some illicit medication."

"Oh, what would make them say that? It's not like you've lost the weight overnight."

"You've got to know the people I work with. When you are starting a diet, they are very supportive. You know the misery loves company crowd, but once you look like you may actually succeed, they get jealous, almost as if you are abandoning them to face their misery alone." When he finished talking, he noticed that Gloria had moved to a chair across from him, and she was smiling and nodding slightly.

"Jealousy could be a good thing, Phil. Maybe you could inspire them to use this approach themselves."

"Are you kidding? I'm very open about what I've done. Some people are even calling me the caloric evangelist." Gloria began to chuckle but stifled it when Phil shot her a baleful glare before continuing. "They call me that because when they ask me about it, I do get excited, and the excitement seems to be contagious until I mention calorie counting. Then, before I mention the part-time nature of the program or how easy and satisfying the full-days are, I get the long faces and the 'I can't be bothered to count calories,' or 'It's too complicated, I don't have time to figure all that out.' When I respond that in the time they take to make a doughnut run, I could have all their caloric numbers figured for them, including what days to use as light vs. full, they just shake their heads and wander away. Probably back to their cubicles to drown their sorrows in high-sugar lattes."

Gloria smiled and said, "Well, as long as they didn't exceed their need, that would be OK." Phil looked at her incredulously, and she laughed out loud. When he didn't join her, she said, "I think I've created a monster. Lighten up, big guy. Maybe you should mention the calorie counting last, after you mention the good stuff. That's what I did with you."

Dourly he responded, "Yes, I suppose you did."

"In all fairness, Phil, you were a bit of a tough nut to crack, and I believe you had to be sold on the idea."

"I know, but I never dismissed it out of hand like some of my erudite colleagues, who think they have the answer to everything because they happen to be math or computer whizzes. You know, I think it's because they see me eat basically like I always did. I even have a doughnut or two once in a while, but what they don't see is that if I do that, I'll skip something else during the day. And it's not like I eat doughnuts every day, but they don't seem to notice that. My indiscretions seem to be the only thing they remember. Sometimes, I feel like they are trying to catch me in a lie."

"You know, Phil, I once had this discussion with my doctor. When I told him of people's reluctance to stick to something that asked for a bare minimum of self-discipline, he pointed out the difficulty he has getting people to take a pill once a day, or, God forbid, two or three times a day. So, don't feel bad, the people who are really ready to try it will listen." Gloria kissed him on the cheek and went back to her homework.

After she left, Phil slipped back into his reverie and decided he should be amused when this claptrap got back to him, after all, who was he anyway to be giving advice. With that resolved, he allowed himself to again savor what he had accomplished, and for the first time since he started this, he could see that the light at the end of the tunnel was not just an optical illusion. The budget proposals and personnel reviews would just have to wait a few more moments.

We have created these two fictitious people to try to show the typical responses and problems most people will encounter, and the typical ways the problems can be surmounted. Once you begin to apply this to your eating habits, you will learn to manipulate it and tailor it to your lifestyle and metabolism. Just follow the basic ideas of limiting your calories three or four days per week and not exceeding your DCN on the other days, thus prioritizing weekly calorie reduction over daily caloric reduction. And, of course, don't forget about exercise.

In the final chapter, we will revisit Phil and Gloria during their maintenance phases. I believe you will be surprised at some of the creative ways you can use this approach to maintain weight and never feel deprived again. To this end, I will introduce the term "legal cheating." I think you will agree it is a very logical, and, dare I say, "cool" way to manage one's weight.

6 | Maintaining The New You

Gloria, Phil, And You Already Know How

If you've ever reached this stage of a diet, you already know that this is the hardest part and the most prone to failure. Some people actually experience a feeling of anxiety when they accomplish this goal, because even before the scale rebounds to zero at their final weigh-in, they realize that they don't really know how to keep a lid on their newfound body weight.

They know they could simply maintain the extraordinary willpower that got them to this goal. But then, wasn't one of the points of this whole endeavor to reach a goal weight and then maintain it WITHOUT extraordinary willpower.

Remember, willpower, in the context of dieting, signifies an internal battle between our biological desires and an idealized image of ourselves. If these two aspects of the psyche cannot come to some type of accord, the biological desires almost always win. In this chapter, we will discuss a strategy to achieve just such an accord.

With this approach, reaching your goal weight should not be cause for anxiety, in fact quite the opposite, because you've been learning all along how to maintain it. Think about it! Each week, you have been dieting down some amount of weight during the light-days, and then holding that weight during the full-days. In other words, you have been dieting down and then maintaining your new weight once per week ever since you started. Now, to remain at your final goal weight, you will observe two simple rules: the first is to eat no more than your full DCN every day, and the second is to maintain your current activity level.

The ability to eat your full DCN every day can produce some interesting options, but before you start, you should be aware that, as with the vacation weeks we discussed above, you <u>may</u> find that after the first week on your full DCN, you gain one or two pounds. This is usually weight as a result of fluid retention. Remember, while you were dieting, a large part of your energy was coming from your body fat. In order to tap into your body fat, you first had to burn muscle glycogen. You can think of this as a form of sugar stored in your muscles to provide quick energy. Glycogen requires water to be stored in the muscles, and when you start eating your full DCN, this glycogen and water will be replenished. You should find that your weight stabilizes after this.

During this final phase, you should weigh yourself regularly to make sure you are not creeping up in weight. The same rules apply for weigh-ins: try to weigh yourself on the same day, first thing in the morning, with the same clothes; but underwear or nude is best. If you find that you are gaining weight, you may need to adjust your DCN calculation, or slightly increase your activity level, or possibly change your activities. Another option you might want to consider is to do one light-day per week: a sort of tune up day if you will. These light-days do not have to be as severe as the light-days you used during the weight loss phase of this program. A reduction of only a few hundred calories from your DCN, one day per week, may be all that is needed to keep you at your goal weight. As with most aspects of this approach, you have more than one option, and which one(s) you use is up to you.

Wait you might be thinking, if you need to lose a pound, the deficit created by one day per week where you eat 500 less than your DCN will take you seven weeks to lose that pound. Strictly speaking, you would be right, except that often when you first notice a little weight gain, much of it is – you already know the answer – fluid, and subtracting 500 calories from one day during the week will often cause a greater weight loss than it might otherwise because of the concomitant fluid loss.

Paradoxically, you may also find that over the weeks and months, you are continuing to lose weight. If this happens, you might want to add a few calories to your DCN. Depending on your activity level, i.e., if you think you are over training, you could also consider cutting back on your training. Under most situations, we would lean toward adding calories to maintain a normal metabolic rate.

Even if it takes a few weeks to find your maintenance DCN, the end result will be worth it, as you should find that you don't have the always-hungry feeling of the chronic dieter and therefore, the tendency to binge at the office party, on weekends, or times of stress etc. is greatly diminished. Remember the accord we spoke of between the biological desires and the idealized image? This is when and how that gets done. We don't suppress the biological desires for the sake of looking good; we just satisfy them without over satisfying them. This agrees with the notion that the correct DCN for you is the one that satisfies your hunger without causing weight gain.

Occasionally though, you might find that you do indeed go over your DCN. While I am not recommending that you overeat, I realize that, being human, we are all prone to the occasional misstep, and sometimes we may get caught up in the moment and, well, you know the rest. Fortunately, this approach offers a very simple way to deal with the infrequent indiscretion. You simply eat less the next day or two. If it is a planned indiscretion, you might do a little pre-emptive dieting and eat lightly a few days beforehand. These two techniques comprise the essence of the term "legal cheating" that was introduced in the previous chapter.

By now, you may be thinking that all this is fine, but you are sick of counting calories and you are wondering if, now that you have reached your goal, there is a way around this necessity. Again, the answer is yes! As part of this learning process, you should have gotten pretty good at gauging when you are full and when you can eat more. By using this feeling and watching the scale, you can pretty much abandon the calorie counter. But wait, why didn't this work before? The answer to that is that before, you didn't have this sense and now because of the weight loss, your stomach has shrunk back to a more normal size. Basically, if you follow these rules, you should be able to maintain your weight without counting every last calorie. The rules are:

➢ Do not eat unless you are hungry.
➢ Eat slowly to allow the full feeling to catch up.
➢ Eat high fiber foods like fruits and vegetables, especially before meals. This will allow time for your blood sugar to rise and blunt your feelings of hunger.

➢ Weigh yourself regularly, not necessarily every day, but no less than once per week, and adjust the amount of food you eat accordingly. So rather than counting calories, you can just pay attention to the amounts of food you eat. For example, if you find that in a given week you have gained a pound or two, the next week, you can simply cut some amount of food from one or more meals. This can be as easy as eating two slices of pizza instead of three, or skipping the fries with a burger, or substituting an apple for a bag of chips with that lunchtime sandwich. If you find that this does not work for you, you can always fall back on counting calories until your internal sense of satiety becomes more accurate.

These rules are simple but powerful, and can be implemented in many ways. In the next section, we will revisit Phil and Gloria to see just some of the ways these rules could be applied in the average person's life.

Gloria Handles Maintenance As Well As Other Issues

In the previous chapter, I mentioned that Gloria had finally reached her goal weight. Let us now backtrack and zoom in on those last few days of dieting and, more importantly, the first days of maintenance to see how she handles it, and what she does to maintain her new "bod".

Gloria rose early that day to do housework. Not because the house was that dirty, but because she wanted to burn a few more calories before her weigh-in. It was October 25th, and she knew today should be the day that she would reach her goal weight. Last week at her weigh-in, the scale said she was a half-pound away, and she found that if she leaned forward a bit, she could actually get it to read her goal weight, but she knew this was cheating. Hopefully, today would be the day she could stand up straight and proud and see the magic number pop up on the face of her electronic scale.

After she cleaned for a while, she noticed that it was getting late so she stopped and took a shower. Later, after drying herself, the moment of truth was at hand. She stepped gingerly on the scale, and in a great flourish, threw the towel on to her bed, and allowed a moment for the numbers to settle. The fluctuating, red numbers finally eased into a steady burn, and Gloria was horrified by what she saw.

According to her scale, she had gained three pounds since last week. Her heart sank, and she sat down on her bed in shock and despair. She would have to wait until next week to actually see her goal weight, even though in terms of actual body fat lost, she was probably at her goal. The salt content in the canned soup and on the crackers, that she had yesterday had been her undoing.

Later that morning, she remembered the soup and crackers and realized these were the most likely causes of her failure, but she was still angry and disappointed, so she decided she would remain on the diet for one more week, just to be sure. When she finally weighed herself the following week, she was at her goal and the next lower number was flickering on the display. She was ecstatic as she realized she could finally start the maintenance phase, meaning she could now eat her full DCN every day and even work on improving her muscle tone.

She is now a little nervous and has actually increased her activity level to sort of hedge her bet. As recommended, she is weighing herself once per week, to make sure she is not slipping into weight gain. After the first week, she is a little dismayed to find that she has indeed gained one pound. She knew to expect this, but secretly hoped it wouldn't happen. For reassurance, she looks in the mirror and is pleased by what she sees. She then decides to try on her smallest jeans to see if they still fit. When she realizes that they fit just as well as last week, she is delighted and, with cautious optimism, resumes the plan.

The following week, she weighs in, finds her weight is steady and breathes a sigh of relief. She is now beginning to focus on other aspects of her life, and food intake is being put in a more proper place. In other words, she is almost on autopilot where her diet is concerned.

She is also finding that the hunger she feels before her usual meal times is indeed satisfied after she eats, and she simply doesn't have that chronic hunger she had before when she was yo-yo dieting. A corollary to this is that, now, when she makes food choices, she makes them more from a place of rationality and less from desperate hunger, so her food choices tend to be better.

After about eight weeks, she notices something completely unexpected during her Friday morning weigh-in. Gloria has lost another pound. She is pleasantly surprised, but a little nonplussed at the weight loss. Gloria thinks back over what she has been doing, and she realizes she has been walking ten minutes per session more than when she was actively losing weight. She decides she would like to remain at this weight, and she could use the time for other things, so she cut ten minutes off of her walks.

A few more pages fly from the calendar, and, all in all, Gloria is now managing her weight pretty well, in fact, she is still one pound under goal, and watching the same number popping up on her digital scale has become quite boring, so without further tedium...

Let's Take A Last Look At Phil

Phil is also doing well, but hasn't quite reached his goal yet. It's not that he isn't staying true to the program; it's just that lately, he's been distracted, and anxious, and he seems to be unable to focus on his work, much less food. His mind is on much bigger things than what he should have for lunch.

Often, he finds himself daydreaming about his past. He examines the triumphs and failures, each in their turn, struggling to read the message contained in their pattern. Finally, he gets up from his chair and walks to the men's lavatory. He feels a little out of breath, and when he sees his reflection in the mirror, he notices a sheen of sweat on his brow, and he feels his heart racing. After he splashes water on his face, he returns to his desk and begins to frantically make phone calls.

A few hours later, Judy Glendenning answered her daughter-in-law's family room phone with a truncated, "Oh hi, Ph..." After one, "Oh good for you," her responses were just answers to a string of interrogatories, like, "No, she's not home yet," "Yes, that sounds fun," and lastly, "OK, I'd be delighted, but you know Gloria and how careful she is, so please make sure you clear it with her first."

Around 5:00 PM the phone rang again; this time it was for Gloria. "Hi Phil. A raise, and a promotion? It's about time they recognized your talent. Dinner tonight? Can't it wait till tomorrow night?" She listened for a while, a look of concern etched on her features and then, "I know, but I had a big lunch today and..." Some more listening and then, "I'm very glad you consider us your family, but that's not going to change between now and tomorrow." Another plea then, "Oh alright, I can see this is really important to you?"

Now that Gloria had acquiesced to Phil's request to go out to dinner with the family, she reflexively ran a rough estimate of calories left to her that day, and she came up with 600, not really enough to indulge in a big dinner. Oddly, a smile brightens her face as she thinks how she might previously have reacted. Ironically, such an offer might have been met with a little anger, and she might have thought that, while it was a nice gesture,

Phil is very aware that she is watching her weight, and he, above all people, should understand when she says she doesn't have enough calories to "pay" for a big dinner.

Now her reaction is quite different because, while most diets would have required strict adherence to whatever their rules are, under her new approach, the rules give her the option to be spontaneous without actually breaching the rules of the system. Remember, as mentioned above, you can make up for the occasional caloric excess by eating light the next day or two, and as it turned out, Gloria would end up doing just that.

While they were getting ready for dinner, Gloria noticed that the kids had dressed up a bit more than their usual jeans and tee shirt. When she asked her daughter why, she said that grand mom had said that Phil was really stoked about this and the restaurant was really nice. Gloria doubted that her mother had used the word "stoked" to describe Phil's enthusiasm, but she too avoided the jeans and opted for a pair of chinos and a pink and pale-blue cotton sweater.

It was exactly mid February, (Hmm, what's that holiday again?) and winter still had the area firmly in its grip as evidenced by the mid teen temperatures extant when Phil arrived to pick them up in his SUV. The ride to the restaurant took almost an hour. This concerned Gloria, as it was a school night for the kids.

The restaurant turned out to be one they had never been to before, and when Gloria saw it, she decided it might have been worth the ride after all. It was located across the street from a ski resort, whose main slope was prominent in the huge picture window in the front of the dining room. Phil held the door as they filed in with the kids first, Gloria second and her mother-in-law last. As they passed him, Judy saw Gloria give Phil an approving nod, and Phil return it with a very slight wry smile of his own. Judy pretended not to notice this and suppressed the urge to smile at Phil's efforts to correct his recent faux pas.

The maitre d' greeted them, and then led them to a large table directly in front of the picture window. Gloria could not stop smiling at the utterly charming ambiance from the rustic décor, to the candles on the table, to the warm muted lighting and of course, the spectacular view of the mountain that seemed to rise up forever into the misty night. When they sat down, she reached under the table and grabbed Phil's hand, squeezed it hard, and smiled a big, broad, silly smile. Phil returned her smile, and she decided that this was indeed the perfect night for this impromptu dinner with the people she loved.

Since Gloria wanted to remain somewhat true to her program, she decided to pick what she knew would be a reasonably priced meal in terms of calories, so she ordered salmon over a bed of wild rice, and allowed herself a glass of their house wine with her meal. If you add up the calories for this meal, you get salmon 180, rice approximately 200, wine is 160, and a dinner salad is roughly 100 with low-fat dressing on the side for a total of 640. Remember, she had 600 left for the day so after eating this, she would have been a little over. If you factor in a 250 – 300 calorie dessert, we are looking at an overage of about 350 calories. Since she has decided to borrow from the next few days, which is perfectly acceptable, this overage is simply no big deal. Gloria smiled as she thought about how nice it was to have the ability to enjoy a nice night out with the family and not have to pay for it with feelings of self-loathing and guilt.

While they were eating, Gloria noticed a few errant snowflakes meandering their way to the ground, as if on tiny pendulums. Since she had been a child, she was always fascinated by the first flakes of a snowfall, and she caught herself involuntarily smiling as she watched them silently piling up on the cold ground.

When they finished their meal and the dishes were being cleared away, the maitre d' walked over to Phil, whispered something in his ear and Phil shook his head affirmatively. Barely a minute later, Gloria's daughter, Jennifer, proclaimed, as only little children can, "Oh cool."

Suddenly, all eyes in the restaurant were trained on the horse-drawn carriage approaching through the cloud of swirling snowflakes. A dapper gentleman wearing a tuxedo and a top hat parked the rig in front of the restaurant, entered through the front door and walked directly to Phil and Gloria's table. Bowing gracefully and removing his top hat in a sweeping arc, he said, "Lady and gentle sir, your carriage awaits."

Phil stood up and offered his hand to Gloria. With tears welling in her eyes, she stood and accepted Phil's hand. As she watched them walk to the carriage, Judy Glendenning had all she could do to fight back her own tears. Jennifer too became misty eyed while Ryan scoffed and wanted to know when he could order dessert.

After the carriage disappeared into the darkness, a woman who appeared a little intoxicated came up to Judy and unabashedly asked if they had just seen the beginnings of a marriage proposal. She could only smile meekly and raise her eyebrows as if to say, 'Your guess is as good as mine.'

The bitter cold caused both Gloria and Phil to shiver as they climbed under the blanket that was on the seat of the carriage. When they were securely in place, the driver gave a quick tug on the reins and made a soft clicking noise with his mouth. The horses instantly reacted and they were off.

The carriage took a small road that led away from the ski area through a field dotted with evergreen trees, and finally wound down into the village below. Phil hadn't said anything yet and seemed more frozen than the snow hitting their faces. Gloria thought about starting the conversation, but she knew this was Phil's moment, and he needed to be the one to take charge.

He finally opened with a little small talk just as they entered the village. "You know, this is fun, but can you imagine having to travel like this all the time."

She suppressed the urge to say something like, "Very romantic observation, Phil. Instead, she said, "I don't know, Phil, it might be nice to slow the world down."

He smiled and said, "I'll remind you of that sentiment the next time your computer freezes."

She laughed and pinched him on the same arm she had been snuggling up to. The levity seemed to break Phil's nervous paralysis, and he began to say what he had really intended. "You know, I can't tell you how happy I've been since I've met you."

She looked deeply into his eyes, turning his muscles into sap, and said in her most demure voice, "Really, Phil, why not?"

He wasn't sure if her playfulness was just her being giddy, or her trying to deflect his advance. He took a deep breath and pushed on. "Gloria, since I've met you, my life just seems to get better and better. It might seem I'm a bit old to say this, but you are the first woman I've ever really loved. You're the first thing I think about when I wake up, and the last thing on my mind when I fall asleep. For God's sake, I have dreams about you probably every other night."

Another impish smile, and she said, "Really, Phil, who do you dream about on the off nights?"

Ignoring her question, he continued, "And I daydream about you way too much at work."

He noticed she was staring at him now, wide-eyed with an exaggerated look of concern, like a parent might do with a frightened child who had just had a nightmare. She said, "That sounds serious. What should we do about it?"

The words echoed through his mind, '*What should we do about it?*' Was that an invitation from her? Was she trying to tell him she was receptive by using the word "we"?

Finally he turned to her, grabbed both her hands in his and thought, damn the torpedoes, just before he blurted, "Well, I know I'd probably sleep better if you would just marry me!"

The night abruptly turned windless and the snow now fell straight down. For a few moments, the silence was broken only by the horses' clip-clop and the wheels crunching through what was now about two inches of snow. Gloria regarded him with a sad smile, squeezed his hands hard enough to make him wince and said, "Screeawk michim blabel."

Oops, sorry, it was at that point that our hidden microphone in the carriage went on the fritz. Maybe it was the snow, or Phil's sappy approach, but something shorted out a circuit or two. Can you imagine asking a woman to marry you so you'll sleep better? We know he meant it tongue-in-cheek, but given the moonless and snowy conditions we just couldn't see if Gloria thought tongue-in-cheek was appropriate at a moment like this. We'll just have to wait until they get back to the restaurant to find out what old Glor said to Phil's clumsy proposal.

B ack at the restaurant, Judy Glendenning stared into a glass of wine she had been nursing. The curious among the patrons had long since gone back to their tables and because the maitre d' had been kind enough to make sure the kids were entertained with coloring books, all she had to do was wait.

She couldn't help sneaking peeks at her watch while the old adage: years fly and seconds crawl, or some such thing reverberated through her mind. At that moment, she could surely vouch for the seconds crawling part. The suspense was killing her.

No matter what happened, it would be bittersweet for her, because, of course, this day would be a watershed in all their lives. If Gloria and Phil got married, she knew her grandkids would get a good stepfather, and although it would make the loss of her son all the more poignant, she knew Gloria would never really forget Hugh. If Gloria said no, or Phil's spine melted, their relationship might just shrivel up and that would be flat out sad because, at least in Judy's estimation, they each represented the best shot at a second chance for each other.

Finally, after close to forty minutes, sounds of sleigh bells and the rhythmic clip-clop of the horse's hooves interrupted her rumination and then, like an apparition, the carriage materialized out of the squall. The sounds had also gotten other people's attention, and Judy couldn't help but notice that it seemed all eyes in the room were gazing through the picture window at the carriage. Seconds, then minutes ticked by before Gloria left the carriage and began walking toward the restaurant, hugging herself against the cold. A few moments later, Phil followed, head bowed.

Jennifer came up behind her grand mom, hugged her and placed her head on Judy's shoulder as she watched her mom and Phil traverse the slippery sidewalk, in single file, from the road to the restaurant's entrance. Hushed whispers and murmurs carried through the restaurant, lamenting poor Phil's failure. Judy heard one man who commented, "Geez, that's tough, and after the whole thing with the carriage and all."

Judy, too, was a bit stunned by what appeared to have happened, but then her eyes narrowed as she focused on something that caught her attention. Within an instant, she began to well up with nascent tears. Jennifer noticed this and asked if she was sad. "No, honey, I think I might be happy." At that moment, Gloria and then Phil disappeared around the corner that blocked the diners' view of the entrance. No one saw Gloria stop and extend her hand for Phil before they entered the restaurant.

Back inside, Jennifer continued her interrogation of her grandmother.

"Why do you think you might be happy, Grandma?"

"Well, I think I'm happy because I think Phil asked your mom to marry him."

"How do you know that, Gram?"

"Did you see his right pant leg?"

Jennifer looked at her nonplussed and said, "I didn't really notice it."

"Well, it was wet."

"So what?"

"The what is that I think your mom might have made Phil go down on one knee to propose."

"You mean like in the old movies?"

"I mean like your dad did when he asked your mom to marry him."

Jennifer shook her head like she understood the significance, but Judy doubted that Jennifer understood that despite his inherent goodness, Phil did not have the sensitivity to have gone down on one knee of his own volition, and that her mother would never make Phil do that if her answer was going to be no. In other words, she just knew Phil was coached. While they were talking, Ryan had walked over, apparently had heard their conversation and issued a terse, "How lame."

Jennifer rolled her eyes at her grandmother before shaking her head and saying, "Men." They both giggled at that and then they heard the front door open and close, and felt a short blast of cold air as Phil and Gloria entered the restaurant. Just then, it seemed a hush fell over the place as if everyone had been caught up in a wave of mass curiosity.

As Phil and Gloria made their way through the foyer and were about to cross the threshold into the dining area, they couldn't help but notice the stares. Intuiting what it was about, Gloria smiled and flashed her new engagement ring, while Phil gave a little thumbs up sign. Instantly, the place erupted in cheers and a spontaneous standing ovation commenced. Gloria curtsied, and Phil gave a self-conscious nod and a wave before they went back to their table.

Judy and Jennifer were also clapping and crying, and they both hugged Gloria before wiping her tears away. Judy then asked why they had left the carriage solo. Gloria responded, a little exasperated, "Oh, Phil thought he lost his cell phone and after he saw me freezing, he said why don't I go in and he would be along in a minute. Now you know me, Mom, I would never have accepted his invitation to leave him on this of all nights, but then it occurred to me that maybe, just maybe." She then gestured to Phil's cell phone sitting innocently on the table next to his silverware. Reflexive head shaking and laughter followed among the three women.

Ryan even seemed to be a little moved, and made it a point to shake Phil's hand. Phil then leaned over and whispered something into the boy's ear that made him smile. Because of the ambient noise in the restaurant, Gloria saw, but couldn't hear what happened, but nonetheless welled up with joy as she thought she had just seen the beginning of real male bonding between her son and his future stepfather. She couldn't imagine what profound thing Phil had whispered to Ryan. Since she, much to her credit, decided it was their secret, she'll never know the profundity Phil whispered was: "Thanks, now where's the cheesecake?" Someone once said that some secrets are better left secrets, and we couldn't agree more.

Later, over dessert, Judy sat down next to Phil and congratulated him on his good fortune, but she couldn't help ribbing him a bit about his style. "Gloria told me you needed a little coaching in the proposing department."

Phil smiled a sheepish grin and said, "I thought I might have blown it there for a while."

Judy put on a mock face of admonition and said, "Marry me and I'll sleep better. Phil, what were you thinking?"

Phil retained his humble grin and said, "Yeah, at first she tsk-tsked me and then she told the driver to stop, and told me to get down on one knee and keep asking until I got it right."

Phil noticed the twinkle in Judy's eye, just before she hugged him. "Take good care of them, Phil, that's all I ask."

"Judy, it will be my great honor and my life's purpose."

Throughout the rest of the night, some of the other diners trickled over to the table to offer congratulations. They also received some unsolicited advice from two "financial planners" who were really life insurance salesmen, and an offer from a local real estate agent to hook them up with a time-share near the ski area. Phil politely tucked their business cards into his breast pocket for later disposal.

So Phil and Gloria are now engaged and that's a good thing for everyone involved. But do you know what the great thing *(at least from our perspective)* about tonight really was? It was that, although Gloria overindulged a bit, she kept a loose count of the overage and calculated that she had exceeded her daily limit by only 700 calories, including dessert and champagne. Two days later, after cutting 350 calories from her daily intake, she was back where she started. No harm done, and the psychological need for a big dinner with the family, not to mention the occasional engagement party, had been squelched.

Since she is a pound light, she could have, just as easily, elected to simply spend a few calories, allowing her weight to creep up a few ounces, or she could have just eaten lightly and stayed within her 600-calorie limit. The decision was hers to make. Some of you might be thinking: *Oh God, she still had to count calories, what a drag*! Is there a way where, for just that one night, she could have said, "Calories be damned?" At this point, many diets would lapse into a lecture about desire and self-discipline, and use figures of speech like "eyes on the prize," or "stay the course," or some other motivational metaphor. In other words, they would offer the facile response and force you to choose between six-pack "abs" and second helpings. The Part-Time Diet Approach does not do that. With this system, the answer to your simple query is a, just as simple, "Yes, *occasionally* you can say calories be damned."

Had Gloria gone out and had a filet mignon munchin', baked potato partakin', cheese cake chompin', chandelier swingin' good time, where she threw away her calorie counter, she could have simply weighed herself the next day and then subtracted some arbitrary number of calories from her DCN over the next few days, until she was back at her goal weight. For example, let's say she totally blew it and consumed an extra 1200 calories for that day. Subtracting 400 calories per day, until she was back at her goal weight, would work fine. Ignoring any water retention issues, it should take three days to return to normal. Subtracting 600 calories for two days would have worked just as well. It's really up to her, and you, if you follow this approach.

You see, once you get to this point, it is really a matter of not letting your weight get out of hand. Damage from one day can easily be rectified over the next day or two or three. Many people think that weight management is a matter of all or nothing, starve or gorge with no middle ground. It should be clear by now that this is not true. Once you reach this stage, weight management is a matter of correcting the small indiscretions as they pop up. Incidentally, most naturally thin people do it this way without really being cognizant of it.

So, as you can now deduce, when it comes to dealing with the vagaries of normal life, Gloria now has bullets in her culinary gun, arrows in her dietary quiver, grenades strapped to her gastronomical bandoleer, and, if that wasn't enough, she even has torpedoes in her nutritional submarine. (Sorry, stupid metaphor overload.)

As mentioned above, this approach works even better for planned extravagances like holiday parties, weddings etc. When you know these occasions are near, you can eat a little less a few days before your shindig, and then pretty much eat what you want at the event. If you employ this method, just try to overlook the envious grumbling of your friends as they wonder why you can eat that way and still stay thin. Gloria has since discovered that this approach works particularly well for impending vacations where she knows she may be eating foods she is not used to.

As we take one last look at Gloria, we find she is smiling just a little more than usual lately. A sense of happiness and accomplishment has pervaded her thinking. One only needs to look at her to discover the reason behind the sense of accomplishment, but the happiness runs a little deeper and is born of the knowledge that for the first time in her adult life, she knows she can really keep this body without the chronic hunger and feelings of self-deprivation she had always associated with a lean physique. She now realizes, a little self-discipline combined with the practical know-how she has gained is the real answer.

Gloria is also very aware that she has diabetes in her family history. She knows she may or may not get it, but she also knows that as long as she follows the program her weight does not have to be a precipitating factor.

She finds this is a very calming and liberating feeling, and she feels that it makes learning to count calories well worth the effort. Having worked with people who have suffered the catastrophic health effects that come with diabetes, we wholeheartedly agree. Now let's go see how Phil is doing.

Phil too, has now reached his goal weight and is now reaping the benefits of his newfound lifestyle. While he is still not in love with working out, Phil considers the results worth the two one-half hour sessions per week. He also continues to walk five days per week. Sometimes, when things are busy at work, he skips his lunchtime walk and transfers it to the weekend. Phil occasionally muses at how flexible this program is, and how he feels he will have to pay for it in another lifetime. Who knew Phil was so karmic?

He also enjoys the same flexibility in his eating program. No, he cannot eat like there is no tomorrow, the way he used to before using this approach, but he, like Gloria, has found that he has very little desire to binge any more. For most people, the bingeing comes after a period of severe caloric deprivation, and since severe caloric deprivation is not part of Phil's world any more, the urge to go overboard with eating simply isn't there.

All that being said, Phil is not a tower of strength, and that is the point. In order to maintain his new body, he doesn't have to be. Just recently, he had to attend a going away party for a fellow employee. It was held at a chain restaurant named for a bird call, where the scantily-clad waitresses kept a steady stream of sexual frustration, hot wings, and mozzarella sticks coming for a solid four hours. Phil's behavior at this bacchanalia was no different than before he started on this program. In other words, he regressed back to his old ways and ate too much, drank too much and had to call Gloria for a ride home. The following Saturday morning, he realized he wasn't feeling well enough to diet, so he just ate his full DCN that day. By Sunday, he was back to his old self and decided he would eat 1000 calories less than his DCN to make up for his sins of Friday night. Monday he did the same, and by Tuesday morning, he was back to his normal weight. That day, while getting ready for work, he smiled as he thought that with a little self-discipline, and taking his eating program one day at a time, he could look and feel good for the rest of his life.

I hope our little peek into the lives of Phil and Gloria has given you an idea of what you can expect from this weight loss plan. Since Phil and Gloria are composites of the experiences of people we have worked with over the years, your experience will not necessarily be exactly the same. As you work through your own weight loss program, you will discover how to use this tool the way it best suits you, and therein lies its power. It does not tell you what to eat or when to eat; it only provides a framework for how much. Basically, for the minor inconvenience of counting calories, you can eat anything you want and have the look you want.

As I said in the beginning of this tome, any calorically restricted diet will produce short-term weight loss. Unfortunately, quick, short-term weight loss often leads to long-term weight gain, increased body fat, and all the attendant health problems that entails. Each failed diet compounds this situation by causing the dieter to lose precious muscle tissue, and consequently, their ability to burn calories, a.k.a., their BMR.

To avoid this, one must focus on slow, sustained loss of body fat and maintenance of muscle tissue. If we are to acknowledge human nature, -as if we have a choice- we must also accept that for long-term success, the dieter must lose or maintain weight in a way that requires the least amount of willpower and offers built in flexibility regarding food choices and number of calories consumed. I believe this system provides all that.

Would it have been better if an absolutely zero effort way to lose all the weight you want, as fast as you want that allowed you to eat until your head popped off had been discovered? Sure, but alas, that grail does not exist. Our bodies are still ancient in that they are designed to store excess energy as body fat against long periods of famine. Since modern culture has provided many of us with the somewhat unnatural situation of having cheap, calorically-dense food, we must find ways to regulate ourselves.

Some people believe science may one day produce a pill that will obviate self-control, or perhaps some day, our bodies will evolve to be naturally thin and store little body fat. Who knows? If life has taught us anything, it is to never say never, but even if that happens, it surely won't happen before this summer, or the next big wedding, or the next class reunion,   so   whattaya   waitin'   for?

APPENDIX A: BMR VALUES

How To Use This Table

Before you look up your BMR, take a moment to scan this table. You will see that each of the three parameters –age, weight, and height- have been incremented differently. In generating this table, I experimented with increments as low as one and as high as 15 for each of these parameters. With increments of one for all parameters, a table just shy of 1400 pages was generated. Because I, and some of my colleagues, thought you might want to, let's say, read this book on an airplane or take it to the beach, this number of pages seemed a bit much.

On the other side of the spectrum, increments of 15 did not produce enough precision, so, after much fiddling, wailing, gnashing of teeth, and comparison, an executive decision to use the increments you see here was made.

Careful perusal of the table will reveal that -☺ Hint: When at any social gathering, just say "careful perusal" of just about anything with a professorial tone, and people will say how, well, professorial you sound. Don't worry, there is no extra charge for this advice- the age parameter is incremented by five, the weight parameter increases by ten, and the height parameter increases by two. You will also notice that male and female BMR calculations have been combined in the same table, rather than generating two tables, another space saver.

To use this table, simply find the age, weight and height that most closely coincide with your own. For example: if you are a 28-year-old female who weighs 138 pounds, and stands five feet two inches tall, you would first find the age closest to yours. In this case it would be 30. Then, you would go to the closest weight, which is 140, and finally read across to the nearest height; in this case, it is exactly 62. Read the number next to bmrF, which in this example is 1407, if you are male, the figure next to bmrM would be your BMR.

What if your weight falls exactly between the increments, say at 135 pounds? Just read the BMR for a person weighing 130 and the BMR for a person weighing 140 and split the difference. For example, if you are a 25-year-old, five feet two inch tall female and

you weigh 135 pounds, you would be halfway between 1387 and
1431, or approximately 1409. That's all there is to it. You are now
ready to apply the activity multiplier.

If our woman from the example above is mildly active, the
multiplier would be 1.375, so 1407 X 1.375 = 1934 calories per day to
maintain her weight. Some of our test readers thought it might be
handy to have this little table here, so, being the really nice guy I am,
I have placed it just before the BMR table for your convenience.
Never forget, this number is just a starting point. It can and probably
will be adjusted up or down as you get to know your caloric needs.
Remember, if all this math does not excite you, the
www.parttimediet.com website will calculate these numbers for you.

 -If you are Sedentary (little or no exercise)
  Calorie-Calculation = BMR X 1.2
 -If you are Lightly Active (light exercise/sports 1-3
  days/week) Calorie-Calculation = BMR X 1.375
 -If you are Moderately Active (moderate exercise/sports
  3-5 days/week) Calorie-Calculation = BMR X 1.55
 -If you are Very Active (hard exercise/sports 6-7
  days/week) Calorie-Calculation = BMR X 1.725
 -If you are Extra Active (very hard daily exercise/sports
  & physical job or 2X day training) Calorie-Calculation
  = BMR X 1.9

BMR TABLE

Age 20

weight 110

hgt 60 bmr<u>M</u> 1376 bmr<u>F</u> 1314 hgt 62 bmr<u>M</u> 1401 bmr<u>F</u> 1323
hgt 64 bmr<u>M</u> 1426 bmr<u>F</u> 1333 hgt 66 bmr<u>M</u> 1452 bmr<u>F</u> 1342
hgt 68 bmr<u>M</u> 1477 bmr<u>F</u> 1351 hgt 70 bmr<u>M</u> 1503 bmr<u>F</u> 1360
hgt 72 bmr<u>M</u> 1528 bmr<u>F</u> 1369 hgt 74 bmr<u>M</u> 1553 bmr<u>F</u> 1378
hgt 76 bmr<u>M</u> 1579 bmr<u>F</u> 1387 hgt 78 bmr<u>M</u> 1604 bmr<u>F</u> 1397

weight 120

hgt 60 bmr<u>M</u> 1438 bmr<u>F</u> 1358 hgt 62 bmr<u>M</u> 1463 bmr<u>F</u> 1367
hgt 64 bmr<u>M</u> 1489 bmr<u>F</u> 1376 hgt 66 bmr<u>M</u> 1514 bmr<u>F</u> 1385
hgt 68 bmr<u>M</u> 1539 bmr<u>F</u> 1394 hgt 70 bmr<u>M</u> 1565 bmr<u>F</u> 1404
hgt 72 bmr<u>M</u> 1590 bmr<u>F</u> 1413 hgt 74 bmr<u>M</u> 1616 bmr<u>F</u> 1422
hgt 76 bmr<u>M</u> 1641 bmr<u>F</u> 1431 hgt 78 bmr<u>M</u> 1666 bmr<u>F</u> 1440

weight 130

hgt 60 bmr<u>M</u> 1500 bmr<u>F</u> 1402 hgt 62 bmr<u>M</u> 1525 bmr<u>F</u> 1411
hgt 64 bmr<u>M</u> 1551 bmr<u>F</u> 1420 hgt 66 bmr<u>M</u> 1576 bmr<u>F</u> 1429
hgt 68 bmr<u>M</u> 1602 bmr<u>F</u> 1438 hgt 70 bmr<u>M</u> 1627 bmr<u>F</u> 1447
hgt 72 bmr<u>M</u> 1652 bmr<u>F</u> 1456 hgt 74 bmr<u>M</u> 1678 bmr<u>F</u> 1465
hgt 76 bmr<u>M</u> 1703 bmr<u>F</u> 1475 hgt 78 bmr<u>M</u> 1729 bmr<u>F</u> 1484

weight 140

hgt 60 bmr<u>M</u> 1562 bmr<u>F</u> 1445 hgt 62 bmr<u>M</u> 1588 bmr<u>F</u> 1454
hgt 64 bmr<u>M</u> 1613 bmr<u>F</u> 1463 hgt 66 bmr<u>M</u> 1638 bmr<u>F</u> 1473
hgt 68 bmr<u>M</u> 1664 bmr<u>F</u> 1482 hgt 70 bmr<u>M</u> 1689 bmr<u>F</u> 1491
hgt 72 bmr<u>M</u> 1715 bmr<u>F</u> 1500 hgt 74 bmr<u>M</u> 1740 bmr<u>F</u> 1509
hgt 76 bmr<u>M</u> 1765 bmr<u>F</u> 1518 hgt 78 bmr<u>M</u> 1791 bmr<u>F</u> 1527

weight 150

hgt 60 bmr<u>M</u> 1624 bmr<u>F</u> 1489 hgt 62 bmr<u>M</u> 1650 bmr<u>F</u> 1498
hgt 64 bmr<u>M</u> 1675 bmr<u>F</u> 1507 hgt 66 bmr<u>M</u> 1701 bmr<u>F</u> 1516
hgt 68 bmr<u>M</u> 1726 bmr<u>F</u> 1525 hgt 70 bmr<u>M</u> 1751 bmr<u>F</u> 1534
hgt 72 bmr<u>M</u> 1777 bmr<u>F</u> 1544 hgt 74 bmr<u>M</u> 1802 bmr<u>F</u> 1553
hgt 76 bmr<u>M</u> 1828 bmr<u>F</u> 1562 hgt 78 bmr<u>M</u> 1853 bmr<u>F</u> 1571

weight 160

hgt 60 bmr<u>M</u> 1687 bmr<u>F</u> 1532   hgt 62 bmr<u>M</u> 1712 bmr<u>F</u> 1541
hgt 64 bmr<u>M</u> 1737 bmr<u>F</u> 1551   hgt 66 bmr<u>M</u> 1763 bmr<u>F</u> 1560
hgt 68 bmr<u>M</u> 1788 bmr<u>F</u> 1569   hgt 70 bmr<u>M</u> 1814 bmr<u>F</u> 1578
hgt 72 bmr<u>M</u> 1839 bmr<u>F</u> 1587   hgt 74 bmr<u>M</u> 1864 bmr<u>F</u> 1596
hgt 76 bmr<u>M</u> 1890 bmr<u>F</u> 1605   hgt 78 bmr<u>M</u> 1915 bmr<u>F</u> 1615

weight 170

hgt 60 bmr<u>M</u> 1749 bmr<u>F</u> 1576   hgt 62 bmr<u>M</u> 1774 bmr<u>F</u> 1585
hgt 64 bmr<u>M</u> 1800 bmr<u>F</u> 1594   hgt 66 bmr<u>M</u> 1825 bmr<u>F</u> 1603
hgt 68 bmr<u>M</u> 1850 bmr<u>F</u> 1612   hgt 70 bmr<u>M</u> 1876 bmr<u>F</u> 1622
hgt 72 bmr<u>M</u> 1901 bmr<u>F</u> 1631   hgt 74 bmr<u>M</u> 1927 bmr<u>F</u> 1640
hgt 76 bmr<u>M</u> 1952 bmr<u>F</u> 1649   hgt 78 bmr<u>M</u> 1977 bmr<u>F</u> 1658

weight 180

hgt 60 bmr<u>M</u> 1811 bmr<u>F</u> 1620   hgt 62 bmr<u>M</u> 1836 bmr<u>F</u> 1629
hgt 64 bmr<u>M</u> 1862 bmr<u>F</u> 1638   hgt 66 bmr<u>M</u> 1887 bmr<u>F</u> 1647
hgt 68 bmr<u>M</u> 1913 bmr<u>F</u> 1656   hgt 70 bmr<u>M</u> 1938 bmr<u>F</u> 1665
hgt 72 bmr<u>M</u> 1963 bmr<u>F</u> 1674   hgt 74 bmr<u>M</u> 1989 bmr<u>F</u> 1683
hgt 76 bmr<u>M</u> 2014 bmr<u>F</u> 1693   hgt 78 bmr<u>M</u> 2040 bmr<u>F</u> 1702

weight 190

hgt 60 bmr<u>M</u> 1873 bmr<u>F</u> 1663   hgt 62 bmr<u>M</u> 1899 bmr<u>F</u> 1672
hgt 64 bmr<u>M</u> 1924 bmr<u>F</u> 1681   hgt 66 bmr<u>M</u> 1949 bmr<u>F</u> 1691
hgt 68 bmr<u>M</u> 1975 bmr<u>F</u> 1700   hgt 70 bmr<u>M</u> 2000 bmr<u>F</u> 1709
hgt 72 bmr<u>M</u> 2026 bmr<u>F</u> 1718   hgt 74 bmr<u>M</u> 2051 bmr<u>F</u> 1727
hgt 76 bmr<u>M</u> 2076 bmr<u>F</u> 1736   hgt 78 bmr<u>M</u> 2102 bmr<u>F</u> 1745

weight 200

hgt 60 bmr<u>M</u> 1935 bmr<u>F</u> 1707   hgt 62 bmr<u>M</u> 1961 bmr<u>F</u> 1716
hgt 64 bmr<u>M</u> 1986 bmr<u>F</u> 1725   hgt 66 bmr<u>M</u> 2012 bmr<u>F</u> 1734
hgt 68 bmr<u>M</u> 2037 bmr<u>F</u> 1743   hgt 70 bmr<u>M</u> 2062 bmr<u>F</u> 1752
hgt 72 bmr<u>M</u> 2088 bmr<u>F</u> 1762   hgt 74 bmr<u>M</u> 2113 bmr<u>F</u> 1771
hgt 76 bmr<u>M</u> 2139 bmr<u>F</u> 1780   hgt 78 bmr<u>M</u> 2164 bmr<u>F</u> 1789

weight 210

hgt 60 bmr<u>M</u> 1998 bmr<u>F</u> 1750   hgt 62 bmr<u>M</u> 2023 bmr<u>F</u> 1759
hgt 64 bmr<u>M</u> 2048 bmr<u>F</u> 1769   hgt 66 bmr<u>M</u> 2074 bmr<u>F</u> 1778
hgt 68 bmr<u>M</u> 2099 bmr<u>F</u> 1787   hgt 70 bmr<u>M</u> 2125 bmr<u>F</u> 1796
hgt 72 bmr<u>M</u> 2150 bmr<u>F</u> 1805   hgt 74 bmr<u>M</u> 2175 bmr<u>F</u> 1814
hgt 76 bmr<u>M</u> 2201 bmr<u>F</u> 1823   hgt 78 bmr<u>M</u> 2226 bmr<u>F</u> 1833

weight 220

hgt 60 bmr<u>M</u> 2060 bmr<u>F</u> 1794   hgt 62 bmr<u>M</u> 2085 bmr<u>F</u> 1803
hgt 64 bmr<u>M</u> 2111 bmr<u>F</u> 1812   hgt 66 bmr<u>M</u> 2136 bmr<u>F</u> 1821
hgt 68 bmr<u>M</u> 2161 bmr<u>F</u> 1830   hgt 70 bmr<u>M</u> 2187 bmr<u>F</u> 1840
hgt 72 bmr<u>M</u> 2212 bmr<u>F</u> 1849   hgt 74 bmr<u>M</u> 2238 bmr<u>F</u> 1858
hgt 76 bmr<u>M</u> 2263 bmr<u>F</u> 1867   hgt 78 bmr<u>M</u> 2288 bmr<u>F</u> 1876

weight 230

hgt 60 bmr<u>M</u> 2122 bmr<u>F</u> 1838   hgt 62 bmr<u>M</u> 2147 bmr<u>F</u> 1847
hgt 64 bmr<u>M</u> 2173 bmr<u>F</u> 1856   hgt 66 bmr<u>M</u> 2198 bmr<u>F</u> 1865
hgt 68 bmr<u>M</u> 2224 bmr<u>F</u> 1874   hgt 70 bmr<u>M</u> 2249 bmr<u>F</u> 1883
hgt 72 bmr<u>M</u> 2274 bmr<u>F</u> 1892   hgt 74 bmr<u>M</u> 2300 bmr<u>F</u> 1901
hgt 76 bmr<u>M</u> 2325 bmr<u>F</u> 1911   hgt 78 bmr<u>M</u> 2351 bmr<u>F</u> 1920

weight 240

hgt 60 bmr<u>M</u> 2184 bmr<u>F</u> 1881   hgt 62 bmr<u>M</u> 2210 bmr<u>F</u> 1890
hgt 64 bmr<u>M</u> 2235 bmr<u>F</u> 1899   hgt 66 bmr<u>M</u> 2260 bmr<u>F</u> 1909
hgt 68 bmr<u>M</u> 2286 bmr<u>F</u> 1918   hgt 70 bmr<u>M</u> 2311 bmr<u>F</u> 1927
hgt 72 bmr<u>M</u> 2337 bmr<u>F</u> 1936   hgt 74 bmr<u>M</u> 2362 bmr<u>F</u> 1945
hgt 76 bmr<u>M</u> 2387 bmr<u>F</u> 1954   hgt 78 bmr<u>M</u> 2413 bmr<u>F</u> 1963

weight 250

hgt 60 bmr<u>M</u> 2246 bmr<u>F</u> 1925   hgt 62 bmr<u>M</u> 2272 bmr<u>F</u> 1934
hgt 64 bmr<u>M</u> 2297 bmr<u>F</u> 1943   hgt 66 bmr<u>M</u> 2323 bmr<u>F</u> 1952
hgt 68 bmr<u>M</u> 2348 bmr<u>F</u> 1961   hgt 70 bmr<u>M</u> 2373 bmr<u>F</u> 1970
hgt 72 bmr<u>M</u> 2399 bmr<u>F</u> 1980   hgt 74 bmr<u>M</u> 2424 bmr<u>F</u> 1989
hgt 76 bmr<u>M</u> 2450 bmr<u>F</u> 1998   hgt 78 bmr<u>M</u> 2475 bmr<u>F</u> 2007

weight 260

hgt 60 bmr<u>M</u> 2309 bmr<u>F</u> 1968   hgt 62 bmr<u>M</u> 2334 bmr<u>F</u> 1977
hgt 64 bmr<u>M</u> 2359 bmr<u>F</u> 1987   hgt 66 bmr<u>M</u> 2385 bmr<u>F</u> 1996
hgt 68 bmr<u>M</u> 2410 bmr<u>F</u> 2005   hgt 70 bmr<u>M</u> 2436 bmr<u>F</u> 2014
hgt 72 bmr<u>M</u> 2461 bmr<u>F</u> 2023   hgt 74 bmr<u>M</u> 2486 bmr<u>F</u> 2032
hgt 76 bmr<u>M</u> 2512 bmr<u>F</u> 2041   hgt 78 bmr<u>M</u> 2537 bmr<u>F</u> 2051

weight 270

hgt 60 bmr<u>M</u> 2371 bmr<u>F</u> 2012   hgt 62 bmr<u>M</u> 2396 bmr<u>F</u> 2021
hgt 64 bmr<u>M</u> 2422 bmr<u>F</u> 2030   hgt 66 bmr<u>M</u> 2447 bmr<u>F</u> 2039
hgt 68 bmr<u>M</u> 2472 bmr<u>F</u> 2048   hgt 70 bmr<u>M</u> 2498 bmr<u>F</u> 2058
hgt 72 bmr<u>M</u> 2523 bmr<u>F</u> 2067   hgt 74 bmr<u>M</u> 2549 bmr<u>F</u> 2076
hgt 76 bmr<u>M</u> 2574 bmr<u>F</u> 2085   hgt 78 bmr<u>M</u> 2599 bmr<u>F</u> 2094

<u>weight</u> 280

hgt 60 bmr<u>M</u> 2433 bmr<u>F</u> 2056 hgt 62 bmr<u>M</u> 2458 bmr<u>F</u> 2065
hgt 64 bmr<u>M</u> 2484 bmr<u>F</u> 2074 hgt 66 bmr<u>M</u> 2509 bmr<u>F</u> 2083
hgt 68 bmr<u>M</u> 2535 bmr<u>F</u> 2092 hgt 70 bmr<u>M</u> 2560 bmr<u>F</u> 2101
hgt 72 bmr<u>M</u> 2585 bmr<u>F</u> 2110 hgt 74 bmr<u>M</u> 2611 bmr<u>F</u> 2119
hgt 76 bmr<u>M</u> 2636 bmr<u>F</u> 2129 hgt 78 bmr<u>M</u> 2662 bmr<u>F</u> 2138

<u>weight</u> 290

hgt 60 bmr<u>M</u> 2495 bmr<u>F</u> 2099 hgt 62 bmr<u>M</u> 2521 bmr<u>F</u> 2108
hgt 64 bmr<u>M</u> 2546 bmr<u>F</u> 2117 hgt 66 bmr<u>M</u> 2571 bmr<u>F</u> 2127
hgt 68 bmr<u>M</u> 2597 bmr<u>F</u> 2136 hgt 70 bmr<u>M</u> 2622 bmr<u>F</u> 2145
hgt 72 bmr<u>M</u> 2648 bmr<u>F</u> 2154 hgt 74 bmr<u>M</u> 2673 bmr<u>F</u> 2163
hgt 76 bmr<u>M</u> 2698 bmr<u>F</u> 2172 hgt 78 bmr<u>M</u> 2724 bmr<u>F</u> 2181

<u>weight</u> 300

hgt 60 bmr<u>M</u> 2557 bmr<u>F</u> 2143 hgt 62 bmr<u>M</u> 2583 bmr<u>F</u> 2152
hgt 64 bmr<u>M</u> 2608 bmr<u>F</u> 2161 hgt 66 bmr<u>M</u> 2634 bmr<u>F</u> 2170
hgt 68 bmr<u>M</u> 2659 bmr<u>F</u> 2179 hgt 70 bmr<u>M</u> 2684 bmr<u>F</u> 2188
hgt 72 bmr<u>M</u> 2710 bmr<u>F</u> 2198 hgt 74 bmr<u>M</u> 2735 bmr<u>F</u> 2207
hgt 76 bmr<u>M</u> 2761 bmr<u>F</u> 2216 hgt 78 bmr<u>M</u> 2786 bmr<u>F</u> 2225

Age 25

<u>weight</u> 110

hgt 60 bmr<u>M</u> 1342 bmr<u>F</u> 1291 hgt 62 bmr<u>M</u> 1367 bmr<u>F</u> 1300
hgt 64 bmr<u>M</u> 1392 bmr<u>F</u> 1309 hgt 66 bmr<u>M</u> 1418 bmr<u>F</u> 1318
hgt 68 bmr<u>M</u> 1443 bmr<u>F</u> 1327 hgt 70 bmr<u>M</u> 1469 bmr<u>F</u> 1337
hgt 72 bmr<u>M</u> 1494 bmr<u>F</u> 1346 hgt 74 bmr<u>M</u> 1519 bmr<u>F</u> 1355
hgt 76 bmr<u>M</u> 1545 bmr<u>F</u> 1364 hgt 78 bmr<u>M</u> 1570 bmr<u>F</u> 1373

<u>weight</u> 120

hgt 60 bmr<u>M</u> 1404 bmr<u>F</u> 1334 hgt 62 bmr<u>M</u> 1429 bmr<u>F</u> 1344
hgt 64 bmr<u>M</u> 1455 bmr<u>F</u> 1353 hgt 66 bmr<u>M</u> 1480 bmr<u>F</u> 1362
hgt 68 bmr<u>M</u> 1505 bmr<u>F</u> 1371 hgt 70 bmr<u>M</u> 1531 bmr<u>F</u> 1380
hgt 72 bmr<u>M</u> 1556 bmr<u>F</u> 1389 hgt 74 bmr<u>M</u> 1582 bmr<u>F</u> 1398
hgt 76 bmr<u>M</u> 1607 bmr<u>F</u> 1408 hgt 78 bmr<u>M</u> 1632 bmr<u>F</u> 1417

<u>weight</u> 130

hgt 60 bmr<u>M</u> 1466 bmr<u>F</u> 1378 hgt 62 bmr<u>M</u> 1491 bmr<u>F</u> 1387
hgt 64 bmr<u>M</u> 1517 bmr<u>F</u> 1396 hgt 66 bmr<u>M</u> 1542 bmr<u>F</u> 1405
hgt 68 bmr<u>M</u> 1568 bmr<u>F</u> 1415 hgt 70 bmr<u>M</u> 1593 bmr<u>F</u> 1424
hgt 72 bmr<u>M</u> 1618 bmr<u>F</u> 1433 hgt 74 bmr<u>M</u> 1644 bmr<u>F</u> 1442
hgt 76 bmr<u>M</u> 1669 bmr<u>F</u> 1451 hgt 78 bmr<u>M</u> 1695 bmr<u>F</u> 1460

weight 140

hgt 60 bmr<u>M</u> 1528 bmr<u>F</u> 1422   hgt 62 bmr<u>M</u> 1554 bmr<u>F</u> 1431
hgt 64 bmr<u>M</u> 1579 bmr<u>F</u> 1440   hgt 66 bmr<u>M</u> 1604 bmr<u>F</u> 1449
hgt 68 bmr<u>M</u> 1630 bmr<u>F</u> 1458   hgt 70 bmr<u>M</u> 1655 bmr<u>F</u> 1467
hgt 72 bmr<u>M</u> 1681 bmr<u>F</u> 1476   hgt 74 bmr<u>M</u> 1706 bmr<u>F</u> 1486
hgt 76 bmr<u>M</u> 1731 bmr<u>F</u> 1495   hgt 78 bmr<u>M</u> 1757 bmr<u>F</u> 1504

weight 150

hgt 60 bmr<u>M</u> 1590 bmr<u>F</u> 1465   hgt 62 bmr<u>M</u> 1616 bmr<u>F</u> 1474
hgt 64 bmr<u>M</u> 1641 bmr<u>F</u> 1483   hgt 66 bmr<u>M</u> 1667 bmr<u>F</u> 1493
hgt 68 bmr<u>M</u> 1692 bmr<u>F</u> 1502   hgt 70 bmr<u>M</u> 1717 bmr<u>F</u> 1511
hgt 72 bmr<u>M</u> 1743 bmr<u>F</u> 1520   hgt 74 bmr<u>M</u> 1768 bmr<u>F</u> 1529
hgt 76 bmr<u>M</u> 1794 bmr<u>F</u> 1538   hgt 78 bmr<u>M</u> 1819 bmr<u>F</u> 1547

weight 160

hgt 60 bmr<u>M</u> 1653 bmr<u>F</u> 1509   hgt 62 bmr<u>M</u> 1678 bmr<u>F</u> 1518
hgt 64 bmr<u>M</u> 1703 bmr<u>F</u> 1527   hgt 66 bmr<u>M</u> 1729 bmr<u>F</u> 1536
hgt 68 bmr<u>M</u> 1754 bmr<u>F</u> 1545   hgt 70 bmr<u>M</u> 1780 bmr<u>F</u> 1555
hgt 72 bmr<u>M</u> 1805 bmr<u>F</u> 1564   hgt 74 bmr<u>M</u> 1830 bmr<u>F</u> 1573
hgt 76 bmr<u>M</u> 1856 bmr<u>F</u> 1582   hgt 78 bmr<u>M</u> 1881 bmr<u>F</u> 1591

weight 170

hgt 60 bmr<u>M</u> 1715 bmr<u>F</u> 1552   hgt 62 bmr<u>M</u> 1740 bmr<u>F</u> 1562
hgt 64 bmr<u>M</u> 1766 bmr<u>F</u> 1571   hgt 66 bmr<u>M</u> 1791 bmr<u>F</u> 1580
hgt 68 bmr<u>M</u> 1816 bmr<u>F</u> 1589   hgt 70 bmr<u>M</u> 1842 bmr<u>F</u> 1598
hgt 72 bmr<u>M</u> 1867 bmr<u>F</u> 1607   hgt 74 bmr<u>M</u> 1893 bmr<u>F</u> 1616
hgt 76 bmr<u>M</u> 1918 bmr<u>F</u> 1626   hgt 78 bmr<u>M</u> 1943 bmr<u>F</u> 1635

weight 180

hgt 60 bmr<u>M</u> 1777 bmr<u>F</u> 1596   hgt 62 bmr<u>M</u> 1802 bmr<u>F</u> 1605
hgt 64 bmr<u>M</u> 1828 bmr<u>F</u> 1614   hgt 66 bmr<u>M</u> 1853 bmr<u>F</u> 1623
hgt 68 bmr<u>M</u> 1879 bmr<u>F</u> 1633   hgt 70 bmr<u>M</u> 1904 bmr<u>F</u> 1642
hgt 72 bmr<u>M</u> 1929 bmr<u>F</u> 1651   hgt 74 bmr<u>M</u> 1955 bmr<u>F</u> 1660
hgt 76 bmr<u>M</u> 1980 bmr<u>F</u> 1669   hgt 78 bmr<u>M</u> 2006 bmr<u>F</u> 1678

weight 190

hgt 60 bmr<u>M</u> 1839 bmr<u>F</u> 1640   hgt 62 hmr<u>M</u> 1865 bmr<u>F</u> 1649
hgt 64 bmr<u>M</u> 1890 bmr<u>F</u> 1658   hgt 66 bmr<u>M</u> 1915 bmr<u>F</u> 1667
hgt 68 bmr<u>M</u> 1941 bmr<u>F</u> 1676   hgt 70 bmr<u>M</u> 1966 bmr<u>F</u> 1685
hgt 72 bmr<u>M</u> 1992 bmr<u>F</u> 1694   hgt 74 bmr<u>M</u> 2017 bmr<u>F</u> 1704
hgt 76 bmr<u>M</u> 2042 bmr<u>F</u> 1713   hgt 78 bmr<u>M</u> 2068 bmr<u>F</u> 1722

weight 200

hgt 60 bmr<u>M</u> 1901 bmr<u>F</u> 1683   hgt 62 bmr<u>M</u> 1927 bmr<u>F</u> 1692
hgt 64 bmr<u>M</u> 1952 bmr<u>F</u> 1701   hgt 66 bmr<u>M</u> 1978 bmr<u>F</u> 1711
hgt 68 bmr<u>M</u> 2003 bmr<u>F</u> 1720   hgt 70 bmr<u>M</u> 2028 bmr<u>F</u> 1729
hgt 72 bmr<u>M</u> 2054 bmr<u>F</u> 1738   hgt 74 bmr<u>M</u> 2079 bmr<u>F</u> 1747
hgt 76 bmr<u>M</u> 2105 bmr<u>F</u> 1756   hgt 78 bmr<u>M</u> 2130 bmr<u>F</u> 1765

weight 210

hgt 60 bmr<u>M</u> 1964 bmr<u>F</u> 1727   hgt 62 bmr<u>M</u> 1989 bmr<u>F</u> 1736
hgt 64 bmr<u>M</u> 2014 bmr<u>F</u> 1745   hgt 66 bmr<u>M</u> 2040 bmr<u>F</u> 1754
hgt 68 bmr<u>M</u> 2065 bmr<u>F</u> 1763   hgt 70 bmr<u>M</u> 2091 bmr<u>F</u> 1773
hgt 72 bmr<u>M</u> 2116 bmr<u>F</u> 1782   hgt 74 bmr<u>M</u> 2141 bmr<u>F</u> 1791
hgt 76 bmr<u>M</u> 2167 bmr<u>F</u> 1800   hgt 78 bmr<u>M</u> 2192 bmr<u>F</u> 1809

weight 220

hgt 60 bmr<u>M</u> 2026 bmr<u>F</u> 1770   hgt 62 bmr<u>M</u> 2051 bmr<u>F</u> 1780
hgt 64 bmr<u>M</u> 2077 bmr<u>F</u> 1789   hgt 66 bmr<u>M</u> 2102 bmr<u>F</u> 1798
hgt 68 bmr<u>M</u> 2127 bmr<u>F</u> 1807   hgt 70 bmr<u>M</u> 2153 bmr<u>F</u> 1816
hgt 72 bmr<u>M</u> 2178 bmr<u>F</u> 1825   hgt 74 bmr<u>M</u> 2204 bmr<u>F</u> 1834
hgt 76 bmr<u>M</u> 2229 bmr<u>F</u> 1844   hgt 78 bmr<u>M</u> 2254 bmr<u>F</u> 1853

weight 230

hgt 60 bmr<u>M</u> 2088 bmr<u>F</u> 1814   hgt 62 bmr<u>M</u> 2113 bmr<u>F</u> 1823
hgt 64 bmr<u>M</u> 2139 bmr<u>F</u> 1832   hgt 66 bmr<u>M</u> 2164 bmr<u>F</u> 1841
hgt 68 bmr<u>M</u> 2190 bmr<u>F</u> 1851   hgt 70 bmr<u>M</u> 2215 bmr<u>F</u> 1860
hgt 72 bmr<u>M</u> 2240 bmr<u>F</u> 1869   hgt 74 bmr<u>M</u> 2266 bmr<u>F</u> 1878
hgt 76 bmr<u>M</u> 2291 bmr<u>F</u> 1887   hgt 78 bmr<u>M</u> 2317 bmr<u>F</u> 1896

weight 240

hgt 60 bmr<u>M</u> 2150 bmr<u>F</u> 1858   hgt 62 bmr<u>M</u> 2176 bmr<u>F</u> 1867
hgt 64 bmr<u>M</u> 2201 bmr<u>F</u> 1876   hgt 66 bmr<u>M</u> 2226 bmr<u>F</u> 1885
hgt 68 bmr<u>M</u> 2252 bmr<u>F</u> 1894   hgt 70 bmr<u>M</u> 2277 bmr<u>F</u> 1903
hgt 72 bmr<u>M</u> 2303 bmr<u>F</u> 1912   hgt 74 bmr<u>M</u> 2328 bmr<u>F</u> 1922
hgt 76 bmr<u>M</u> 2353 bmr<u>F</u> 1931   hgt 78 bmr<u>M</u> 2379 bmr<u>F</u> 1940

weight 250

hgt 60 bmr<u>M</u> 2212 bmr<u>F</u> 1901   hgt 62 bmr<u>M</u> 2238 bmr<u>F</u> 1910
hgt 64 bmr<u>M</u> 2263 bmr<u>F</u> 1919   hgt 66 bmr<u>M</u> 2289 bmr<u>F</u> 1929
hgt 68 bmr<u>M</u> 2314 bmr<u>F</u> 1938   hgt 70 bmr<u>M</u> 2339 bmr<u>F</u> 1947
hgt 72 bmr<u>M</u> 2365 bmr<u>F</u> 1956   hgt 74 bmr<u>M</u> 2390 bmr<u>F</u> 1965
hgt 76 bmr<u>M</u> 2416 bmr<u>F</u> 1974   hgt 78 bmr<u>M</u> 2441 bmr<u>F</u> 1983

weight 260

hgt 60 bmr<u>M</u> 2275 bmr<u>F</u> 1945   hgt 62 bmr<u>M</u> 2300 bmr<u>F</u> 1954
hgt 64 bmr<u>M</u> 2325 bmr<u>F</u> 1963   hgt 66 bmr<u>M</u> 2351 bmr<u>F</u> 1972
hgt 68 bmr<u>M</u> 2376 bmr<u>F</u> 1981   hgt 70 bmr<u>M</u> 2402 bmr<u>F</u> 1991
hgt 72 bmr<u>M</u> 2427 bmr<u>F</u> 2000   hgt 74 bmr<u>M</u> 2452 bmr<u>F</u> 2009
hgt 76 bmr<u>M</u> 2478 bmr<u>F</u> 2018   hgt 78 bmr<u>M</u> 2503 bmr<u>F</u> 2027

weight 270

hgt 60 bmr<u>M</u> 2337 bmr<u>F</u> 1988   hgt 62 bmr<u>M</u> 2362 bmr<u>F</u> 1998
hgt 64 bmr<u>M</u> 2388 bmr<u>F</u> 2007   hgt 66 bmr<u>M</u> 2413 bmr<u>F</u> 2016
hgt 68 bmr<u>M</u> 2438 bmr<u>F</u> 2025   hgt 70 bmr<u>M</u> 2464 bmr<u>F</u> 2034
hgt 72 bmr<u>M</u> 2489 bmr<u>F</u> 2043   hgt 74 bmr<u>M</u> 2515 bmr<u>F</u> 2052
hgt 76 bmr<u>M</u> 2540 bmr<u>F</u> 2062   hgt 78 bmr<u>M</u> 2565 bmr<u>F</u> 2071

weight 280

hgt 60 bmr<u>M</u> 2399 bmr<u>F</u> 2032   hgt 62 bmr<u>M</u> 2424 bmr<u>F</u> 2041
hgt 64 bmr<u>M</u> 2450 bmr<u>F</u> 2050   hgt 66 bmr<u>M</u> 2475 bmr<u>F</u> 2059
hgt 68 bmr<u>M</u> 2501 bmr<u>F</u> 2069   hgt 70 bmr<u>M</u> 2526 bmr<u>F</u> 2078
hgt 72 bmr<u>M</u> 2551 bmr<u>F</u> 2087   hgt 74 bmr<u>M</u> 2577 bmr<u>F</u> 2096
hgt 76 bmr<u>M</u> 2602 bmr<u>F</u> 2105   hgt 78 bmr<u>M</u> 2628 bmr<u>F</u> 2114

weight 290

hgt 60 bmr<u>M</u> 2461 bmr<u>F</u> 2076   hgt 62 bmr<u>M</u> 2487 bmr<u>F</u> 2085
hgt 64 bmr<u>M</u> 2512 bmr<u>F</u> 2094   hgt 66 bmr<u>M</u> 2537 bmr<u>F</u> 2103
hgt 68 bmr<u>M</u> 2563 bmr<u>F</u> 2112   hgt 70 bmr<u>M</u> 2588 bmr<u>F</u> 2121
hgt 72 bmr<u>M</u> 2614 bmr<u>F</u> 2130   hgt 74 bmr<u>M</u> 2639 bmr<u>F</u> 2140
hgt 76 bmr<u>M</u> 2664 bmr<u>F</u> 2149   hgt 78 bmr<u>M</u> 2690 bmr<u>F</u> 2158

weight 300

hgt 60 bmr<u>M</u> 2523 bmr<u>F</u> 2119   hgt 62 bmr<u>M</u> 2549 bmr<u>F</u> 2128
hgt 64 bmr<u>M</u> 2574 bmr<u>F</u> 2137   hgt 66 bmr<u>M</u> 2600 bmr<u>F</u> 2147
hgt 68 bmr<u>M</u> 2625 bmr<u>F</u> 2156   hgt 70 bmr<u>M</u> 2650 bmr<u>F</u> 2165
hgt 72 bmr<u>M</u> 2676 bmr<u>F</u> 2174   hgt 74 bmr<u>M</u> 2701 bmr<u>F</u> 2183
hgt 76 bmr<u>M</u> 2727 bmr<u>F</u> 2192   hgt 78 bmr<u>M</u> 2752 bmr<u>F</u> 2201

Age 30

weight 110

hgt 60 bmr<u>M</u> 1308 bmr<u>F</u> 1267   hgt 62 bmr<u>M</u> 1333 bmr<u>F</u> 1276
hgt 64 bmr<u>M</u> 1358 bmr<u>F</u> 1286   hgt 66 bmr<u>M</u> 1384 bmr<u>F</u> 1295
hgt 68 bmr<u>M</u> 1409 bmr<u>F</u> 1304   hgt 70 bmr<u>M</u> 1435 bmr<u>F</u> 1313
hgt 72 bmr<u>M</u> 1460 bmr<u>F</u> 1322   hgt 74 bmr<u>M</u> 1485 bmr<u>F</u> 1331
hgt 76 bmr<u>M</u> 1511 bmr<u>F</u> 1340   hgt 78 bmr<u>M</u> 1536 bmr<u>F</u> 1350

weight 120

hgt 60 bmr<u>M</u> 1370 bmr<u>F</u> 1311   hgt 62 bmr<u>M</u> 1395 bmr<u>F</u> 1320
hgt 64 bmr<u>M</u> 1421 bmr<u>F</u> 1329   hgt 66 bmr<u>M</u> 1446 bmr<u>F</u> 1338
hgt 68 bmr<u>M</u> 1471 bmr<u>F</u> 1347   hgt 70 bmr<u>M</u> 1497 bmr<u>F</u> 1357
hgt 72 bmr<u>M</u> 1522 bmr<u>F</u> 1366   hgt 74 bmr<u>M</u> 1548 bmr<u>F</u> 1375
hgt 76 bmr<u>M</u> 1573 bmr<u>F</u> 1384   hgt 78 bmr<u>M</u> 1598 bmr<u>F</u> 1393

weight 130

hgt 60 bmr<u>M</u> 1432 bmr<u>F</u> 1355   hgt 62 bmr<u>M</u> 1457 bmr<u>F</u> 1364
hgt 64 bmr<u>M</u> 1483 bmr<u>F</u> 1373   hgt 66 bmr<u>M</u> 1508 bmr<u>F</u> 1382
hgt 68 bmr<u>M</u> 1534 bmr<u>F</u> 1391   hgt 70 bmr<u>M</u> 1559 bmr<u>F</u> 1400
hgt 72 bmr<u>M</u> 1584 bmr<u>F</u> 1409   hgt 74 bmr<u>M</u> 1610 bmr<u>F</u> 1418
hgt 76 bmr<u>M</u> 1635 bmr<u>F</u> 1428   hgt 78 bmr<u>M</u> 1661 bmr<u>F</u> 1437

weight 140

hgt 60 bmr<u>M</u> 1494 bmr<u>F</u> 1398   hgt 62 bmr<u>M</u> 1520 bmr<u>F</u> 1407
hgt 64 bmr<u>M</u> 1545 bmr<u>F</u> 1416   hgt 66 bmr<u>M</u> 1570 bmr<u>F</u> 1426
hgt 68 bmr<u>M</u> 1596 bmr<u>F</u> 1435   hgt 70 bmr<u>M</u> 1621 bmr<u>F</u> 1444
hgt 72 bmr<u>M</u> 1647 bmr<u>F</u> 1453   hgt 74 bmr<u>M</u> 1672 bmr<u>F</u> 1462
hgt 76 bmr<u>M</u> 1697 bmr<u>F</u> 1471   hgt 78 bmr<u>M</u> 1723 bmr<u>F</u> 1480

weight 150

hgt 60 bmr<u>M</u> 1556 bmr<u>F</u> 1442   hgt 62 bmr<u>M</u> 1582 bmr<u>F</u> 1451
hgt 64 bmr<u>M</u> 1607 bmr<u>F</u> 1460   hgt 66 bmr<u>M</u> 1633 bmr<u>F</u> 1469
hgt 68 bmr<u>M</u> 1658 bmr<u>F</u> 1478   hgt 70 bmr<u>M</u> 1683 bmr<u>F</u> 1487
hgt 72 bmr<u>M</u> 1709 bmr<u>F</u> 1497   hgt 74 bmr<u>M</u> 1734 bmr<u>F</u> 1506
hgt 76 bmr<u>M</u> 1760 bmr<u>F</u> 1515   hgt 78 bmr<u>M</u> 1785 bmr<u>F</u> 1524

weight 160

hgt 60 bmr<u>M</u> 1619 bmr<u>F</u> 1485   hgt 62 bmr<u>M</u> 1644 bmr<u>F</u> 1494
hgt 64 bmr<u>M</u> 1669 bmr<u>F</u> 1504   hgt 66 bmr<u>M</u> 1695 bmr<u>F</u> 1513
hgt 68 bmr<u>M</u> 1720 bmr<u>F</u> 1522   hgt 70 bmr<u>M</u> 1746 bmr<u>F</u> 1531
hgt 72 bmr<u>M</u> 1771 bmr<u>F</u> 1540   hgt 74 bmr<u>M</u> 1796 bmr<u>F</u> 1549
hgt 76 bmr<u>M</u> 1822 bmr<u>F</u> 1558   hgt 78 bmr<u>M</u> 1847 bmr<u>F</u> 1568

weight 170

hgt 60 bmr<u>M</u> 1681 bmr<u>F</u> 1529   hgt 62 bmr<u>M</u> 1706 bmr<u>F</u> 1538
hgt 64 bmr<u>M</u> 1732 bmr<u>F</u> 1547   hgt 66 bmr<u>M</u> 1757 bmr<u>F</u> 1556
hgt 68 bmr<u>M</u> 1782 bmr<u>F</u> 1565   hgt 70 bmr<u>M</u> 1808 bmr<u>F</u> 1575
hgt 72 bmr<u>M</u> 1833 bmr<u>F</u> 1584   hgt 74 bmr<u>M</u> 1859 bmr<u>F</u> 1593
hgt 76 bmr<u>M</u> 1884 bmr<u>F</u> 1602   hgt 78 bmr<u>M</u> 1909 bmr<u>F</u> 1611

weight 180

hgt 60 bmr<u>M</u> 1743 bmr<u>F</u> 1573 hgt 62 bmr<u>M</u> 1768 bmr<u>F</u> 1582
hgt 64 bmr<u>M</u> 1794 bmr<u>F</u> 1591 hgt 66 bmr<u>M</u> 1819 bmr<u>F</u> 1600
hgt 68 bmr<u>M</u> 1845 bmr<u>F</u> 1609 hgt 70 bmr<u>M</u> 1870 bmr<u>F</u> 1618
hgt 72 bmr<u>M</u> 1895 bmr<u>F</u> 1627 hgt 74 bmr<u>M</u> 1921 bmr<u>F</u> 1636
hgt 76 bmr<u>M</u> 1946 bmr<u>F</u> 1646 hgt 78 bmr<u>M</u> 1972 bmr<u>F</u> 1655

weight 190

hgt 60 bmr<u>M</u> 1805 bmr<u>F</u> 1616 hgt 62 bmr<u>M</u> 1831 bmr<u>F</u> 1625
hgt 64 bmr<u>M</u> 1856 bmr<u>F</u> 1634 hgt 66 bmr<u>M</u> 1881 bmr<u>F</u> 1644
hgt 68 bmr<u>M</u> 1907 bmr<u>F</u> 1653 hgt 70 bmr<u>M</u> 1932 bmr<u>F</u> 1662
hgt 72 bmr<u>M</u> 1958 bmr<u>F</u> 1671 hgt 74 bmr<u>M</u> 1983 bmr<u>F</u> 1680
hgt 76 bmr<u>M</u> 2008 bmr<u>F</u> 1689 hgt 78 bmr<u>M</u> 2034 bmr<u>F</u> 1698

weight 200

hgt 60 bmr<u>M</u> 1867 bmr<u>F</u> 1660 hgt 62 bmr<u>M</u> 1893 bmr<u>F</u> 1669
hgt 64 bmr<u>M</u> 1918 bmr<u>F</u> 1678 hgt 66 bmr<u>M</u> 1944 bmr<u>F</u> 1687
hgt 68 bmr<u>M</u> 1969 bmr<u>F</u> 1696 hgt 70 bmr<u>M</u> 1994 bmr<u>F</u> 1705
hgt 72 bmr<u>M</u> 2020 bmr<u>F</u> 1715 hgt 74 bmr<u>M</u> 2045 bmr<u>F</u> 1724
hgt 76 bmr<u>M</u> 2071 bmr<u>F</u> 1733 hgt 78 bmr<u>M</u> 2096 bmr<u>F</u> 1742

weight 210

hgt 60 bmr<u>M</u> 1930 bmr<u>F</u> 1703 hgt 62 bmr<u>M</u> 1955 bmr<u>F</u> 1712
hgt 64 bmr<u>M</u> 1980 bmr<u>F</u> 1722 hgt 66 bmr<u>M</u> 2006 bmr<u>F</u> 1731
hgt 68 bmr<u>M</u> 2031 bmr<u>F</u> 1740 hgt 70 bmr<u>M</u> 2057 bmr<u>F</u> 1749
hgt 72 bmr<u>M</u> 2082 bmr<u>F</u> 1758 hgt 74 bmr<u>M</u> 2107 bmr<u>F</u> 1767
hgt 76 bmr<u>M</u> 2133 bmr<u>F</u> 1776 hgt 78 bmr<u>M</u> 2158 bmr<u>F</u> 1786

weight 220

hgt 60 bmr<u>M</u> 1992 bmr<u>F</u> 1747 hgt 62 bmr<u>M</u> 2017 bmr<u>F</u> 1756
hgt 64 bmr<u>M</u> 2043 bmr<u>F</u> 1765 hgt 66 bmr<u>M</u> 2068 bmr<u>F</u> 1774
hgt 68 bmr<u>M</u> 2093 bmr<u>F</u> 1783 hgt 70 bmr<u>M</u> 2119 bmr<u>F</u> 1793
hgt 72 bmr<u>M</u> 2144 bmr<u>F</u> 1802 hgt 74 bmr<u>M</u> 2170 bmr<u>F</u> 1811
hgt 76 bmr<u>M</u> 2195 bmr<u>F</u> 1820 hgt 78 bmr<u>M</u> 2220 bmr<u>F</u> 1829

weight 230

hgt 60 bmr<u>M</u> 2054 bmr<u>F</u> 1791 hgt 62 bmr<u>M</u> 2079 bmr<u>F</u> 1800
hgt 64 bmr<u>M</u> 2105 bmr<u>F</u> 1809 hgt 66 bmr<u>M</u> 2130 bmr<u>F</u> 1818
hgt 68 bmr<u>M</u> 2156 bmr<u>F</u> 1827 hgt 70 bmr<u>M</u> 2181 bmr<u>F</u> 1836
hgt 72 bmr<u>M</u> 2206 bmr<u>F</u> 1845 hgt 74 bmr<u>M</u> 2232 bmr<u>F</u> 1854
hgt 76 bmr<u>M</u> 2257 bmr<u>F</u> 1864 hgt 78 bmr<u>M</u> 2283 bmr<u>F</u> 1873

<u>weight</u> 240

hgt 60	bmr<u>M</u> 2116	bmr<u>F</u> 1834	hgt 62	bmr<u>M</u> 2142	bmr<u>F</u> 1843
hgt 64	bmr<u>M</u> 2167	bmr<u>F</u> 1852	hgt 66	bmr<u>M</u> 2192	bmr<u>F</u> 1862
hgt 68	bmr<u>M</u> 2218	bmr<u>F</u> 1871	hgt 70	bmr<u>M</u> 2243	bmr<u>F</u> 1880
hgt 72	bmr<u>M</u> 2269	bmr<u>F</u> 1889	hgt 74	bmr<u>M</u> 2294	bmr<u>F</u> 1898
hgt 76	bmr<u>M</u> 2319	bmr<u>F</u> 1907	hgt 78	bmr<u>M</u> 2345	bmr<u>F</u> 1916

<u>weight</u> 250

hgt 60	bmr<u>M</u> 2178	bmr<u>F</u> 1878	hgt 62	bmr<u>M</u> 2204	bmr<u>F</u> 1887
hgt 64	bmr<u>M</u> 2229	bmr<u>F</u> 1896	hgt 66	bmr<u>M</u> 2255	bmr<u>F</u> 1905
hgt 68	bmr<u>M</u> 2280	bmr<u>F</u> 1914	hgt 70	bmr<u>M</u> 2305	bmr<u>F</u> 1923
hgt 72	bmr<u>M</u> 2331	bmr<u>F</u> 1933	hgt 74	bmr<u>M</u> 2356	bmr<u>F</u> 1942
hgt 76	bmr<u>M</u> 2382	bmr<u>F</u> 1951	hgt 78	bmr<u>M</u> 2407	bmr<u>F</u> 1960

<u>weight</u> 260

hgt 60	bmr<u>M</u> 2241	bmr<u>F</u> 1921	hgt 62	bmr<u>M</u> 2266	bmr<u>F</u> 1930
hgt 64	bmr<u>M</u> 2291	bmr<u>F</u> 1940	hgt 66	bmr<u>M</u> 2317	bmr<u>F</u> 1949
hgt 68	bmr<u>M</u> 2342	bmr<u>F</u> 1958	hgt 70	bmr<u>M</u> 2368	bmr<u>F</u> 1967
hgt 72	bmr<u>M</u> 2393	bmr<u>F</u> 1976	hgt 74	bmr<u>M</u> 2418	bmr<u>F</u> 1985
hgt 76	bmr<u>M</u> 2444	bmr<u>F</u> 1994	hgt 78	bmr<u>M</u> 2469	bmr<u>F</u> 2004

<u>weight</u> 270

hgt 60	bmr<u>M</u> 2303	bmr<u>F</u> 1965	hgt 62	bmr<u>M</u> 2328	bmr<u>F</u> 1974
hgt 64	bmr<u>M</u> 2354	bmr<u>F</u> 1983	hgt 66	bmr<u>M</u> 2379	bmr<u>F</u> 1992
hgt 68	bmr<u>M</u> 2404	bmr<u>F</u> 2001	hgt 70	bmr<u>M</u> 2430	bmr<u>F</u> 2011
hgt 72	bmr<u>M</u> 2455	bmr<u>F</u> 2020	hgt 74	bmr<u>M</u> 2481	bmr<u>F</u> 2029
hgt 76	bmr<u>M</u> 2506	bmr<u>F</u> 2038	hgt 78	bmr<u>M</u> 2531	bmr<u>F</u> 2047

<u>weight</u> 280

hgt 60	bmr<u>M</u> 2365	bmr<u>F</u> 2009	hgt 62	bmr<u>M</u> 2390	bmr<u>F</u> 2018
hgt 64	bmr<u>M</u> 2416	bmr<u>F</u> 2027	hgt 66	bmr<u>M</u> 2441	bmr<u>F</u> 2036
hgt 68	bmr<u>M</u> 2467	bmr<u>F</u> 2045	hgt 70	bmr<u>M</u> 2492	bmr<u>F</u> 2054
hgt 72	bmr<u>M</u> 2517	bmr<u>F</u> 2063	hgt 74	bmr<u>M</u> 2543	bmr<u>F</u> 2072
hgt 76	bmr<u>M</u> 2568	bmr<u>F</u> 2082	hgt 78	bmr<u>M</u> 2594	bmr<u>F</u> 2091

<u>weight</u> 290

hgt 60	bmr<u>M</u> 2427	bmr<u>F</u> 2052	hgt 62	bmr<u>M</u> 2453	bmr<u>F</u> 2061
hgt 64	bmr<u>M</u> 2478	bmr<u>F</u> 2070	hgt 66	bmr<u>M</u> 2503	bmr<u>F</u> 2080
hgt 68	bmr<u>M</u> 2529	bmr<u>F</u> 2089	hgt 70	bmr<u>M</u> 2554	bmr<u>F</u> 2098
hgt 72	bmr<u>M</u> 2580	bmr<u>F</u> 2107	hgt 74	bmr<u>M</u> 2605	bmr<u>F</u> 2116
hgt 76	bmr<u>M</u> 2630	bmr<u>F</u> 2125	hgt 78	bmr<u>M</u> 2656	bmr<u>F</u> 2134

weight 300

hgt 60 bmrM 2489 bmrF 2096 hgt 62 bmrM 2515 bmrF 2105
hgt 64 bmrM 2540 bmrF 2114 hgt 66 bmrM 2566 bmrF 2123
hgt 68 bmrM 2591 bmrF 2132 hgt 70 bmrM 2616 bmrF 2141
hgt 72 bmrM 2642 bmrF 2151 hgt 74 bmrM 2667 bmrF 2160
hgt 76 bmrM 2693 bmrF 2169 hgt 78 bmrM 2718 bmrF 2178

Age 35

weight 110

hgt 60 bmrM 1274 bmrF 1244 hgt 62 bmrM 1299 bmrF 1253
hgt 64 bmrM 1324 bmrF 1262 hgt 66 bmrM 1350 bmrF 1271
hgt 68 bmrM 1375 bmrF 1280 hgt 70 bmrM 1401 bmrF 1290
hgt 72 bmrM 1426 bmrF 1299 hgt 74 bmrM 1451 bmrF 1308
hgt 76 bmrM 1477 bmrF 1317 hgt 78 bmrM 1502 bmrF 1326

weight 120

hgt 60 bmrM 1336 bmrF 1287 hgt 62 bmrM 1361 bmrF 1297
hgt 64 bmrM 1387 bmrF 1306 hgt 66 bmrM 1412 bmrF 1315
hgt 68 bmrM 1437 bmrF 1324 hgt 70 bmrM 1463 bmrF 1333
hgt 72 bmrM 1488 bmrF 1342 hgt 74 bmrM 1514 bmrF 1351
hgt 76 bmrM 1539 bmrF 1361 hgt 78 bmrM 1564 bmrF 1370

weight 130

hgt 60 bmrM 1398 bmrF 1331 hgt 62 bmrM 1423 bmrF 1340
hgt 64 bmrM 1449 bmrF 1349 hgt 66 bmrM 1474 bmrF 1358
hgt 68 bmrM 1500 bmrF 1368 hgt 70 bmrM 1525 bmrF 1377
hgt 72 bmrM 1550 bmrF 1386 hgt 74 bmrM 1576 bmrF 1395
hgt 76 bmrM 1601 bmrF 1404 hgt 78 bmrM 1627 bmrF 1413

weight 140

hgt 60 bmrM 1460 bmrF 1375 hgt 62 bmrM 1486 bmrF 1384
hgt 64 bmrM 1511 bmrF 1393 hgt 66 bmrM 1536 bmrF 1402
hgt 68 bmrM 1562 bmrF 1411 hgt 70 bmrM 1587 bmrF 1420
hgt 72 bmrM 1613 bmrF 1429 hgt 74 bmrM 1638 bmrF 1439
hgt 76 bmrM 1663 bmrF 1448 hgt 78 bmrM 1689 bmrF 1457

weight 150

hgt 60 bmrM 1522 bmrF 1418 hgt 62 bmrM 1548 bmrF 1427
hgt 64 bmrM 1573 bmrF 1436 hgt 66 bmrM 1599 bmrF 1446
hgt 68 bmrM 1624 bmrF 1455 hgt 70 bmrM 1649 bmrF 1464
hgt 72 bmrM 1675 bmrF 1473 hgt 74 bmrM 1700 bmrF 1482
hgt 76 bmrM 1726 bmrF 1491 hgt 78 bmrM 1751 bmrF 1500

weight 160

hgt 60 bmr<u>M</u> 1585 bmr<u>F</u> 1462   hgt 62 bmr<u>M</u> 1610 bmr<u>F</u> 1471
hgt 64 bmr<u>M</u> 1635 bmr<u>F</u> 1480   hgt 66 bmr<u>M</u> 1661 bmr<u>F</u> 1489
hgt 68 bmr<u>M</u> 1686 bmr<u>F</u> 1498   hgt 70 bmr<u>M</u> 1712 bmr<u>F</u> 1508
hgt 72 bmr<u>M</u> 1737 bmr<u>F</u> 1517   hgt 74 bmr<u>M</u> 1762 bmr<u>F</u> 1526
hgt 76 bmr<u>M</u> 1788 bmr<u>F</u> 1535   hgt 78 bmr<u>M</u> 1813 bmr<u>F</u> 1545

weight 170

hgt 60 bmr<u>M</u> 1647 bmr<u>F</u> 1505   hgt 62 bmr<u>M</u> 1672 bmr<u>F</u> 1515
hgt 64 bmr<u>M</u> 1698 bmr<u>F</u> 1524   hgt 66 bmr<u>M</u> 1723 bmr<u>F</u> 1533
hgt 68 bmr<u>M</u> 1748 bmr<u>F</u> 1542   hgt 70 bmr<u>M</u> 1774 bmr<u>F</u> 1551
hgt 72 bmr<u>M</u> 1799 bmr<u>F</u> 1560   hgt 74 bmr<u>M</u> 1825 bmr<u>F</u> 1569
hgt 76 bmr<u>M</u> 1850 bmr<u>F</u> 1579   hgt 78 bmr<u>M</u> 1875 bmr<u>F</u> 1588

weight 180

hgt 60 bmr<u>M</u> 1709 bmr<u>F</u> 1549   hgt 62 bmr<u>M</u> 1734 bmr<u>F</u> 1558
hgt 64 bmr<u>M</u> 1760 bmr<u>F</u> 1567   hgt 66 bmr<u>M</u> 1785 bmr<u>F</u> 1576
hgt 68 bmr<u>M</u> 1811 bmr<u>F</u> 1586   hgt 70 bmr<u>M</u> 1836 bmr<u>F</u> 1595
hgt 72 bmr<u>M</u> 1861 bmr<u>F</u> 1604   hgt 74 bmr<u>M</u> 1887 bmr<u>F</u> 1613
hgt 76 bmr<u>M</u> 1912 bmr<u>F</u> 1622   hgt 78 bmr<u>M</u> 1938 bmr<u>F</u> 1631

weight 190

hgt 60 bmr<u>M</u> 1771 bmr<u>F</u> 1593   hgt 62 bmr<u>M</u> 1797 bmr<u>F</u> 1602
hgt 64 bmr<u>M</u> 1822 bmr<u>F</u> 1611   hgt 66 bmr<u>M</u> 1847 bmr<u>F</u> 1620
hgt 68 bmr<u>M</u> 1873 bmr<u>F</u> 1629   hgt 70 bmr<u>M</u> 1898 bmr<u>F</u> 1638
hgt 72 bmr<u>M</u> 1924 bmr<u>F</u> 1647   hgt 74 bmr<u>M</u> 1949 bmr<u>F</u> 1657
hgt 76 bmr<u>M</u> 1974 bmr<u>F</u> 1666   hgt 78 bmr<u>M</u> 2000 bmr<u>F</u> 1675

weight 200

hgt 60 bmr<u>M</u> 1833 bmr<u>F</u> 1636   hgt 62 bmr<u>M</u> 1859 bmr<u>F</u> 1645
hgt 64 bmr<u>M</u> 1884 bmr<u>F</u> 1654   hgt 66 bmr<u>M</u> 1910 bmr<u>F</u> 1664
hgt 68 bmr<u>M</u> 1935 bmr<u>F</u> 1673   hgt 70 bmr<u>M</u> 1960 bmr<u>F</u> 1682
hgt 72 bmr<u>M</u> 1986 bmr<u>F</u> 1691   hgt 74 bmr<u>M</u> 2011 bmr<u>F</u> 1700
hgt 76 bmr<u>M</u> 2037 bmr<u>F</u> 1709   hgt 78 bmr<u>M</u> 2062 bmr<u>F</u> 1718

weight 210

hgt 60 bmr<u>M</u> 1896 bmr<u>F</u> 1680   hgt 62 bmr<u>M</u> 1921 bmr<u>F</u> 1689
hgt 64 bmr<u>M</u> 1946 bmr<u>F</u> 1698   hgt 66 bmr<u>M</u> 1972 bmr<u>F</u> 1707
hgt 68 bmr<u>M</u> 1997 bmr<u>F</u> 1716   hgt 70 bmr<u>M</u> 2023 bmr<u>F</u> 1726
hgt 72 bmr<u>M</u> 2048 bmr<u>F</u> 1735   hgt 74 bmr<u>M</u> 2073 bmr<u>F</u> 1744
hgt 76 bmr<u>M</u> 2099 bmr<u>F</u> 1753   hgt 78 bmr<u>M</u> 2124 bmr<u>F</u> 1762

<u>weight</u> 220

hgt 60 bmr<u>M</u> 1958 bmr<u>F</u> 1723 hgt 62 bmr<u>M</u> 1983 bmr<u>F</u> 1733
hgt 64 bmr<u>M</u> 2009 bmr<u>F</u> 1742 hgt 66 bmr<u>M</u> 2034 bmr<u>F</u> 1751
hgt 68 bmr<u>M</u> 2059 bmr<u>F</u> 1760 hgt 70 bmr<u>M</u> 2085 bmr<u>F</u> 1769
hgt 72 bmr<u>M</u> 2110 bmr<u>F</u> 1778 hgt 74 bmr<u>M</u> 2136 bmr<u>F</u> 1787
hgt 76 bmr<u>M</u> 2161 bmr<u>F</u> 1797 hgt 78 bmr<u>M</u> 2186 bmr<u>F</u> 1806

<u>weight</u> 230

hgt 60 bmr<u>M</u> 2020 bmr<u>F</u> 1767 hgt 62 bmr<u>M</u> 2045 bmr<u>F</u> 1776
hgt 64 bmr<u>M</u> 2071 bmr<u>F</u> 1785 hgt 66 bmr<u>M</u> 2096 bmr<u>F</u> 1794
hgt 68 bmr<u>M</u> 2122 bmr<u>F</u> 1804 hgt 70 bmr<u>M</u> 2147 bmr<u>F</u> 1813
hgt 72 bmr<u>M</u> 2172 bmr<u>F</u> 1822 hgt 74 bmr<u>M</u> 2198 bmr<u>F</u> 1831
hgt 76 bmr<u>M</u> 2223 bmr<u>F</u> 1840 hgt 78 bmr<u>M</u> 2249 bmr<u>F</u> 1849

<u>weight</u> 240

hgt 60 bmr<u>M</u> 2082 bmr<u>F</u> 1811 hgt 62 bmr<u>M</u> 2108 bmr<u>F</u> 1820
hgt 64 bmr<u>M</u> 2133 bmr<u>F</u> 1829 hgt 66 bmr<u>M</u> 2158 bmr<u>F</u> 1838
hgt 68 bmr<u>M</u> 2184 bmr<u>F</u> 1847 hgt 70 bmr<u>M</u> 2209 bmr<u>F</u> 1856
hgt 72 bmr<u>M</u> 2235 bmr<u>F</u> 1865 hgt 74 bmr<u>M</u> 2260 bmr<u>F</u> 1875
hgt 76 bmr<u>M</u> 2285 bmr<u>F</u> 1884 hgt 78 bmr<u>M</u> 2311 bmr<u>F</u> 1893

<u>weight</u> 250

hgt 60 bmr<u>M</u> 2144 bmr<u>F</u> 1854 hgt 62 bmr<u>M</u> 2170 bmr<u>F</u> 1863
hgt 64 bmr<u>M</u> 2195 bmr<u>F</u> 1872 hgt 66 bmr<u>M</u> 2221 bmr<u>F</u> 1882
hgt 68 bmr<u>M</u> 2246 bmr<u>F</u> 1891 hgt 70 bmr<u>M</u> 2271 bmr<u>F</u> 1900
hgt 72 bmr<u>M</u> 2297 bmr<u>F</u> 1909 hgt 74 bmr<u>M</u> 2322 bmr<u>F</u> 1918
hgt 76 bmr<u>M</u> 2348 bmr<u>F</u> 1927 hgt 78 bmr<u>M</u> 2373 bmr<u>F</u> 1936

<u>weight</u> 260

hgt 60 bmr<u>M</u> 2207 bmr<u>F</u> 1898 hgt 62 bmr<u>M</u> 2232 bmr<u>F</u> 1907
hgt 64 bmr<u>M</u> 2257 bmr<u>F</u> 1916 hgt 66 bmr<u>M</u> 2283 bmr<u>F</u> 1925
hgt 68 bmr<u>M</u> 2308 bmr<u>F</u> 1934 hgt 70 bmr<u>M</u> 2334 bmr<u>F</u> 1944
hgt 72 bmr<u>M</u> 2359 bmr<u>F</u> 1953 hgt 74 bmr<u>M</u> 2384 bmr<u>F</u> 1962
hgt 76 bmr<u>M</u> 2410 bmr<u>F</u> 1971 hgt 78 bmr<u>M</u> 2435 bmr<u>F</u> 1980

<u>weight</u> 270

hgt 60 bmr<u>M</u> 2269 bmr<u>F</u> 1941 hgt 62 bmr<u>M</u> 2294 bmr<u>F</u> 1951
hgt 64 bmr<u>M</u> 2320 bmr<u>F</u> 1960 hgt 66 bmr<u>M</u> 2345 bmr<u>F</u> 1969
hgt 68 bmr<u>M</u> 2370 bmr<u>F</u> 1978 hgt 70 bmr<u>M</u> 2396 bmr<u>F</u> 1987
hgt 72 bmr<u>M</u> 2421 bmr<u>F</u> 1996 hgt 74 bmr<u>M</u> 2447 bmr<u>F</u> 2005
hgt 76 bmr<u>M</u> 2472 bmr<u>F</u> 2015 hgt 78 bmr<u>M</u> 2497 bmr<u>F</u> 2024

<u>weight</u> 280

hgt 60 bmr<u>M</u> 2331 bmr<u>F</u> 1985   hgt 62 bmr<u>M</u> 2356 bmr<u>F</u> 1994
hgt 64 bmr<u>M</u> 2382 bmr<u>F</u> 2003   hgt 66 bmr<u>M</u> 2407 bmr<u>F</u> 2012
hgt 68 bmr<u>M</u> 2433 bmr<u>F</u> 2022   hgt 70 bmr<u>M</u> 2458 bmr<u>F</u> 2031
hgt 72 bmr<u>M</u> 2483 bmr<u>F</u> 2040   hgt 74 bmr<u>M</u> 2509 bmr<u>F</u> 2049
hgt 76 bmr<u>M</u> 2534 bmr<u>F</u> 2058   hgt 78 bmr<u>M</u> 2560 bmr<u>F</u> 2067

<u>weight</u> 290

hgt 60 bmr<u>M</u> 2393 bmr<u>F</u> 2029   hgt 62 bmr<u>M</u> 2419 bmr<u>F</u> 2038
hgt 64 bmr<u>M</u> 2444 bmr<u>F</u> 2047   hgt 66 bmr<u>M</u> 2469 bmr<u>F</u> 2056
hgt 68 bmr<u>M</u> 2495 bmr<u>F</u> 2065   hgt 70 bmr<u>M</u> 2520 bmr<u>F</u> 2074
hgt 72 bmr<u>M</u> 2546 bmr<u>F</u> 2083   hgt 74 bmr<u>M</u> 2571 bmr<u>F</u> 2093
hgt 76 bmr<u>M</u> 2596 bmr<u>F</u> 2102   hgt 78 bmr<u>M</u> 2622 bmr<u>F</u> 2111

<u>weight</u> 300

hgt 60 bmr<u>M</u> 2455 bmr<u>F</u> 2072   hgt 62 bmr<u>M</u> 2481 bmr<u>F</u> 2081
hgt 64 bmr<u>M</u> 2506 bmr<u>F</u> 2090   hgt 66 bmr<u>M</u> 2532 bmr<u>F</u> 2100
hgt 68 bmr<u>M</u> 2557 bmr<u>F</u> 2109   hgt 70 bmr<u>M</u> 2582 bmr<u>F</u> 2118
hgt 72 bmr<u>M</u> 2608 bmr<u>F</u> 2127   hgt 74 bmr<u>M</u> 2633 bmr<u>F</u> 2136
hgt 76 bmr<u>M</u> 2659 bmr<u>F</u> 2145   hgt 78 bmr<u>M</u> 2684 bmr<u>F</u> 2154

Age 40

<u>weight</u> 110

hgt 60 bmr<u>M</u> 1240 bmr<u>F</u> 1220   hgt 62 bmr<u>M</u> 1265 bmr<u>F</u> 1229
hgt 64 bmr<u>M</u> 1290 bmr<u>F</u> 1239   hgt 66 bmr<u>M</u> 1316 bmr<u>F</u> 1248
hgt 68 bmr<u>M</u> 1341 bmr<u>F</u> 1257   hgt 70 bmr<u>M</u> 1367 bmr<u>F</u> 1266
hgt 72 bmr<u>M</u> 1392 bmr<u>F</u> 1275   hgt 74 bmr<u>M</u> 1417 bmr<u>F</u> 1284
hgt 76 bmr<u>M</u> 1443 bmr<u>F</u> 1293   hgt 78 bmr<u>M</u> 1468 bmr<u>F</u> 1303

<u>weight</u> 120

hgt 60 bmr<u>M</u> 1302 bmr<u>F</u> 1264   hgt 62 bmr<u>M</u> 1327 bmr<u>F</u> 1273
hgt 64 bmr<u>M</u> 1353 bmr<u>F</u> 1282   hgt 66 bmr<u>M</u> 1378 bmr<u>F</u> 1291
hgt 68 bmr<u>M</u> 1403 bmr<u>F</u> 1300   hgt 70 bmr<u>M</u> 1429 bmr<u>F</u> 1310
hgt 72 bmr<u>M</u> 1454 bmr<u>F</u> 1319   hgt 74 bmr<u>M</u> 1480 bmr<u>F</u> 1328
hgt 76 bmr<u>M</u> 1505 bmr<u>F</u> 1337   hgt 78 bmr<u>M</u> 1530 bmr<u>F</u> 1346

<u>weight</u> 130

hgt 60 bmr<u>M</u> 1364 bmr<u>F</u> 1308   hgt 62 bmr<u>M</u> 1389 bmr<u>F</u> 1317
hgt 64 bmr<u>M</u> 1415 bmr<u>F</u> 1326   hgt 66 bmr<u>M</u> 1440 bmr<u>F</u> 1335
hgt 68 bmr<u>M</u> 1466 bmr<u>F</u> 1344   hgt 70 bmr<u>M</u> 1491 bmr<u>F</u> 1353
hgt 72 bmr<u>M</u> 1516 bmr<u>F</u> 1362   hgt 74 bmr<u>M</u> 1542 bmr<u>F</u> 1371
hgt 76 bmr<u>M</u> 1567 bmr<u>F</u> 1381   hgt 78 bmr<u>M</u> 1593 bmr<u>F</u> 1390

weight 140
hgt 60 bmr<u>M</u> 1426 bmr<u>F</u> 1351 hgt 62 bmr<u>M</u> 1452 bmr<u>F</u> 1360
hgt 64 bmr<u>M</u> 1477 bmr<u>F</u> 1369 hgt 66 bmr<u>M</u> 1502 bmr<u>F</u> 1379
hgt 68 bmr<u>M</u> 1528 bmr<u>F</u> 1388 hgt 70 bmr<u>M</u> 1553 bmr<u>F</u> 1397
hgt 72 bmr<u>M</u> 1579 bmr<u>F</u> 1406 hgt 74 bmr<u>M</u> 1604 bmr<u>F</u> 1415
hgt 76 bmr<u>M</u> 1629 bmr<u>F</u> 1424 hgt 78 bmr<u>M</u> 1655 bmr<u>F</u> 1433

weight 150
hgt 60 bmr<u>M</u> 1488 bmr<u>F</u> 1395 hgt 62 bmr<u>M</u> 1514 bmr<u>F</u> 1404
hgt 64 bmr<u>M</u> 1539 bmr<u>F</u> 1413 hgt 66 bmr<u>M</u> 1565 bmr<u>F</u> 1422
hgt 68 bmr<u>M</u> 1590 bmr<u>F</u> 1431 hgt 70 bmr<u>M</u> 1615 bmr<u>F</u> 1440
hgt 72 bmr<u>M</u> 1641 bmr<u>F</u> 1450 hgt 74 bmr<u>M</u> 1666 bmr<u>F</u> 1459
hgt 76 bmr<u>M</u> 1692 bmr<u>F</u> 1468 hgt 78 bmr<u>M</u> 1717 bmr<u>F</u> 1477

weight 160
hgt 60 bmr<u>M</u> 1551 bmr<u>F</u> 1438 hgt 62 bmr<u>M</u> 1576 bmr<u>F</u> 1447
hgt 64 bmr<u>M</u> 1601 bmr<u>F</u> 1457 hgt 66 bmr<u>M</u> 1627 bmr<u>F</u> 1466
hgt 68 bmr<u>M</u> 1652 bmr<u>F</u> 1475 hgt 70 bmr<u>M</u> 1678 bmr<u>F</u> 1484
hgt 72 bmr<u>M</u> 1703 bmr<u>F</u> 1493 hgt 74 bmr<u>M</u> 1728 bmr<u>F</u> 1502
hgt 76 bmr<u>M</u> 1754 bmr<u>F</u> 1511 hgt 78 bmr<u>M</u> 1779 bmr<u>F</u> 1521

weight 170
hgt 60 bmr<u>M</u> 1613 bmr<u>F</u> 1482 hgt 62 bmr<u>M</u> 1638 bmr<u>F</u> 1491
hgt 64 bmr<u>M</u> 1664 bmr<u>F</u> 1500 hgt 66 bmr<u>M</u> 1689 bmr<u>F</u> 1509
hgt 68 bmr<u>M</u> 1714 bmr<u>F</u> 1518 hgt 70 bmr<u>M</u> 1740 bmr<u>F</u> 1528
hgt 72 bmr<u>M</u> 1765 bmr<u>F</u> 1537 hgt 74 bmr<u>M</u> 1791 bmr<u>F</u> 1546
hgt 76 bmr<u>M</u> 1816 bmr<u>F</u> 1555 hgt 78 bmr<u>M</u> 1841 bmr<u>F</u> 1564

weight 180
hgt 60 bmr<u>M</u> 1675 bmr<u>F</u> 1526 hgt 62 bmr<u>M</u> 1700 bmr<u>F</u> 1535
hgt 64 bmr<u>M</u> 1726 bmr<u>F</u> 1544 hgt 66 bmr<u>M</u> 1751 bmr<u>F</u> 1553
hgt 68 bmr<u>M</u> 1777 bmr<u>F</u> 1562 hgt 70 bmr<u>M</u> 1802 bmr<u>T</u> 1571
hgt 72 bmr<u>M</u> 1827 bmr<u>F</u> 1580 hgt 74 bmr<u>M</u> 1853 bmr<u>F</u> 1589
hgt 76 bmr<u>M</u> 1878 bmr<u>F</u> 1599 hgt 78 bmr<u>M</u> 1904 bmr<u>F</u> 1608

weight 190
hgt 60 bmr<u>M</u> 1737 bmr<u>F</u> 1569 hgt 62 bmr<u>M</u> 1763 bmr<u>F</u> 1578
hgt 64 bmr<u>M</u> 1788 bmr<u>F</u> 1587 hgt 66 bmr<u>M</u> 1813 bmr<u>F</u> 1597
hgt 68 bmr<u>M</u> 1839 bmr<u>F</u> 1606 hgt 70 bmr<u>M</u> 1864 bmr<u>F</u> 1615
hgt 72 bmr<u>M</u> 1890 bmr<u>F</u> 1624 hgt 74 bmr<u>M</u> 1915 bmr<u>F</u> 1633
hgt 76 bmr<u>M</u> 1940 bmr<u>F</u> 1642 hgt 78 bmr<u>M</u> 1966 bmr<u>F</u> 1651

<u>weight</u> 200

hgt 60 bmr<u>M</u> 1799 bmr<u>F</u> 1613   hgt 62 bmr<u>M</u> 1825 bmr<u>F</u> 1622
hgt 64 bmr<u>M</u> 1850 bmr<u>F</u> 1631   hgt 66 bmr<u>M</u> 1876 bmr<u>F</u> 1640
hgt 68 bmr<u>M</u> 1901 bmr<u>F</u> 1649   hgt 70 bmr<u>M</u> 1926 bmr<u>F</u> 1658
hgt 72 bmr<u>M</u> 1952 bmr<u>F</u> 1668   hgt 74 bmr<u>M</u> 1977 bmr<u>F</u> 1677
hgt 76 bmr<u>M</u> 2003 bmr<u>F</u> 1686   hgt 78 bmr<u>M</u> 2028 bmr<u>F</u> 1695

<u>weight</u> 210

hgt 60 bmr<u>M</u> 1862 bmr<u>F</u> 1656   hgt 62 bmr<u>M</u> 1887 bmr<u>F</u> 1665
hgt 64 bmr<u>M</u> 1912 bmr<u>F</u> 1675   hgt 66 bmr<u>M</u> 1938 bmr<u>F</u> 1684
hgt 68 bmr<u>M</u> 1963 bmr<u>F</u> 1693   hgt 70 bmr<u>M</u> 1989 bmr<u>F</u> 1702
hgt 72 bmr<u>M</u> 2014 bmr<u>F</u> 1711   hgt 74 bmr<u>M</u> 2039 bmr<u>F</u> 1720
hgt 76 bmr<u>M</u> 2065 bmr<u>F</u> 1729   hgt 78 bmr<u>M</u> 2090 bmr<u>F</u>

<u>weight</u> 220

hgt 60 bmr<u>M</u> 1924 bmr<u>F</u> 1700   hgt 62 bmr<u>M</u> 1949 bmr<u>F</u> 1709
hgt 64 bmr<u>M</u> 1975 bmr<u>F</u> 1718   hgt 66 bmr<u>M</u> 2000 bmr<u>F</u> 1727
hgt 68 bmr<u>M</u> 2025 bmr<u>F</u> 1736   hgt 70 bmr<u>M</u> 2051 bmr<u>F</u> 1746
hgt 72 bmr<u>M</u> 2076 bmr<u>F</u> 1755   hgt 74 bmr<u>M</u> 2102 bmr<u>F</u> 1764
hgt 76 bmr<u>M</u> 2127 bmr<u>F</u> 1773   hgt 78 bmr<u>M</u> 2152 bmr<u>F</u> 1782

<u>weight</u> 230

hgt 60 bmr<u>M</u> 1986 bmr<u>F</u> 1744   hgt 62 bmr<u>M</u> 2011 bmr<u>F</u> 1753
hgt 64 bmr<u>M</u> 2037 bmr<u>F</u> 1762   hgt 66 bmr<u>M</u> 2062 bmr<u>F</u> 1771
hgt 68 bmr<u>M</u> 2088 bmr<u>F</u> 1780   hgt 70 bmr<u>M</u> 2113 bmr<u>F</u> 1789
hgt 72 bmr<u>M</u> 2138 bmr<u>F</u> 1798   hgt 74 bmr<u>M</u> 2164 bmr<u>F</u> 1807
hgt 76 bmr<u>M</u> 2189 bmr<u>F</u> 1817   hgt 78 bmr<u>M</u> 2215 bmr<u>F</u> 1826

<u>weight</u> 240

hgt 60 bmr<u>M</u> 2048 bmr<u>F</u> 1787   hgt 62 bmr<u>M</u> 2074 bmr<u>F</u> 1796
hgt 64 bmr<u>M</u> 2099 bmr<u>F</u> 1805   hgt 66 bmr<u>M</u> 2124 bmr<u>F</u> 1815
hgt 68 bmr<u>M</u> 2150 bmr<u>F</u> 1824   hgt 70 bmr<u>M</u> 2175 bmr<u>F</u> 1833
hgt 72 bmr<u>M</u> 2201 bmr<u>F</u> 1842   hgt 74 bmr<u>M</u> 2226 bmr<u>F</u> 1851
hgt 76 bmr<u>M</u> 2251 bmr<u>F</u> 1860   hgt 78 bmr<u>M</u> 2277 bmr<u>F</u> 1869

<u>weight</u> 250

hgt 60 bmr<u>M</u> 2110 bmr<u>F</u> 1831   hgt 62 bmr<u>M</u> 2136 bmr<u>F</u> 1840
hgt 64 bmr<u>M</u> 2161 bmr<u>F</u> 1849   hgt 66 bmr<u>M</u> 2187 bmr<u>F</u> 1858
hgt 68 bmr<u>M</u> 2212 bmr<u>F</u> 1867   hgt 70 bmr<u>M</u> 2237 bmr<u>F</u> 1876
hgt 72 bmr<u>M</u> 2263 bmr<u>F</u> 1886   hgt 74 bmr<u>M</u> 2288 bmr<u>F</u> 1895
hgt 76 bmr<u>M</u> 2314 bmr<u>F</u> 1904   hgt 78 bmr<u>M</u> 2339 bmr<u>F</u> 1913

weight 260

hgt 60 bmr<u>M</u> 2173 bmr<u>F</u> 1874 hgt 62 bmr<u>M</u> 2198 bmr<u>F</u> 1883
hgt 64 bmr<u>M</u> 2223 bmr<u>F</u> 1893 hgt 66 bmr<u>M</u> 2249 bmr<u>F</u> 1902
hgt 68 bmr<u>M</u> 2274 bmr<u>F</u> 1911 hgt 70 bmr<u>M</u> 2300 bmr<u>F</u> 1920
hgt 72 bmr<u>M</u> 2325 bmr<u>F</u> 1929 hgt 74 bmr<u>M</u> 2350 bmr<u>F</u> 1938
hgt 76 bmr<u>M</u> 2376 bmr<u>F</u> 1947 hgt 78 bmr<u>M</u> 2401 bmr<u>F</u> 1957

weight 270

hgt 60 bmr<u>M</u> 2235 bmr<u>F</u> 1918 hgt 62 bmr<u>M</u> 2260 bmr<u>F</u> 1927
hgt 64 bmr<u>M</u> 2286 bmr<u>F</u> 1936 hgt 66 bmr<u>M</u> 2311 bmr<u>F</u> 1945
hgt 68 bmr<u>M</u> 2336 bmr<u>F</u> 1954 hgt 70 bmr<u>M</u> 2362 bmr<u>F</u> 1964
hgt 72 bmr<u>M</u> 2387 bmr<u>F</u> 1973 hgt 74 bmr<u>M</u> 2413 bmr<u>F</u> 1982
hgt 76 bmr<u>M</u> 2438 bmr<u>F</u> 1991 hgt 78 bmr<u>M</u> 2463 bmr<u>F</u> 2000

weight 280

hgt 60 bmr<u>M</u> 2297 bmr<u>F</u> 1962 hgt 62 bmr<u>M</u> 2322 bmr<u>F</u> 1971
hgt 64 bmr<u>M</u> 2348 bmr<u>F</u> 1980 hgt 66 bmr<u>M</u> 2373 bmr<u>F</u> 1989
hgt 68 bmr<u>M</u> 2399 bmr<u>F</u> 1998 hgt 70 bmr<u>M</u> 2424 bmr<u>F</u> 2007
hgt 72 bmr<u>M</u> 2449 bmr<u>F</u> 2016 hgt 74 bmr<u>M</u> 2475 bmr<u>F</u> 2025
hgt 76 bmr<u>M</u> 2500 bmr<u>F</u> 2035 hgt 78 bmr<u>M</u> 2526 bmr<u>F</u> 2044

weight 290

hgt 60 bmr<u>M</u> 2359 bmr<u>F</u> 2005 hgt 62 bmr<u>M</u> 2385 bmr<u>F</u> 2014
hgt 64 bmr<u>M</u> 2410 bmr<u>F</u> 2023 hgt 66 bmr<u>M</u> 2435 bmr<u>F</u> 2033
hgt 68 bmr<u>M</u> 2461 bmr<u>F</u> 2042 hgt 70 bmr<u>M</u> 2486 bmr<u>F</u> 2051
hgt 72 bmr<u>M</u> 2512 bmr<u>F</u> 2060 hgt 74 bmr<u>M</u> 2537 bmr<u>F</u> 2069
hgt 76 bmr<u>M</u> 2562 bmr<u>F</u> 2078 hgt 78 bmr<u>M</u> 2588 bmr<u>F</u> 2087

weight 300

hgt 60 bmr<u>M</u> 2421 bmr<u>F</u> 2049 hgt 62 bmr<u>M</u> 2447 bmr<u>F</u> 2058
hgt 64 bmr<u>M</u> 2472 bmr<u>F</u> 2067 hgt 66 bmr<u>M</u> 2498 bmr<u>F</u> 2076
hgt 68 bmr<u>M</u> 2523 bmr<u>F</u> 2085 hgt 70 bmr<u>M</u> 2548 bmr<u>F</u> 2094
hgt 72 bmr<u>M</u> 2574 bmr<u>F</u> 2104 hgt 74 bmr<u>M</u> 2599 bmr<u>F</u> 2113
hgt 76 bmr<u>M</u> 2625 bmr<u>F</u> 2122 hgt 78 bmr<u>M</u> 2650 bmr<u>F</u> 2131

Age 45

weight 110

hgt 60 bmr<u>M</u> 1206 bmr<u>F</u> 1197 hgt 62 bmr<u>M</u> 1231 bmr<u>F</u> 1206
hgt 64 bmr<u>M</u> 1256 bmr<u>F</u> 1215 hgt 66 bmr<u>M</u> 1282 bmr<u>F</u> 1224
hgt 68 bmr<u>M</u> 1307 bmr<u>F</u> 1233 hgt 70 bmr<u>M</u> 1333 bmr<u>F</u> 1243
hgt 72 bmr<u>M</u> 1358 bmr<u>F</u> 1252 hgt 74 bmr<u>M</u> 1383 bmr<u>F</u> 1261
hgt 76 bmr<u>M</u> 1409 bmr<u>F</u> 1270 hgt 78 bmr<u>M</u> 1434 bmr<u>F</u> 1279

weight 120

hgt 60 bmr<u>M</u> 1268 bmr<u>F</u> 1240   hgt 62 bmr<u>M</u> 1293 bmr<u>F</u> 1250
hgt 64 bmr<u>M</u> 1319 bmr<u>F</u> 1259   hgt 66 bmr<u>M</u> 1344 bmr<u>F</u> 1268
hgt 68 bmr<u>M</u> 1369 bmr<u>F</u> 1277   hgt 70 bmr<u>M</u> 1395 bmr<u>F</u> 1286
hgt 72 bmr<u>M</u> 1420 bmr<u>F</u> 1295   hgt 74 bmr<u>M</u> 1446 bmr<u>F</u> 1304
hgt 76 bmr<u>M</u> 1471 bmr<u>F</u> 1314   hgt 78 bmr<u>M</u> 1496 bmr<u>F</u> 1323

weight 130

hgt 60 bmr<u>M</u> 1330 bmr<u>F</u> 1284   hgt 62 bmr<u>M</u> 1355 bmr<u>F</u> 1293
hgt 64 bmr<u>M</u> 1381 bmr<u>F</u> 1302   hgt 66 bmr<u>M</u> 1406 bmr<u>F</u> 1311
hgt 68 bmr<u>M</u> 1432 bmr<u>F</u> 1321   hgt 70 bmr<u>M</u> 1457 bmr<u>F</u> 1330
hgt 72 bmr<u>M</u> 1482 bmr<u>F</u> 1339   hgt 74 bmr<u>M</u> 1508 bmr<u>F</u> 1348
hgt 76 bmr<u>M</u> 1533 bmr<u>F</u> 1357   hgt 78 bmr<u>M</u> 1559 bmr<u>F</u> 1366

weight 140

hgt 60 bmr<u>M</u> 1392 bmr<u>F</u> 1328   hgt 62 bmr<u>M</u> 1418 bmr<u>F</u> 1337
hgt 64 bmr<u>M</u> 1443 bmr<u>F</u> 1346   hgt 66 bmr<u>M</u> 1468 bmr<u>F</u> 1355
hgt 68 bmr<u>M</u> 1494 bmr<u>F</u> 1364   hgt 70 bmr<u>M</u> 1519 bmr<u>F</u> 1373
hgt 72 bmr<u>M</u> 1545 bmr<u>F</u> 1382   hgt 74 bmr<u>M</u> 1570 bmr<u>F</u> 1392
hgt 76 bmr<u>M</u> 1595 bmr<u>F</u> 1401   hgt 78 bmr<u>M</u> 1621 bmr<u>F</u> 1410

weight 150

hgt 60 bmr<u>M</u> 1454 bmr<u>F</u> 1371   hgt 62 bmr<u>M</u> 1480 bmr<u>F</u> 1380
hgt 64 bmr<u>M</u> 1505 bmr<u>F</u> 1389   hgt 66 bmr<u>M</u> 1531 bmr<u>F</u> 1399
hgt 68 bmr<u>M</u> 1556 bmr<u>F</u> 1408   hgt 70 bmr<u>M</u> 1581 bmr<u>F</u> 1417
hgt 72 bmr<u>M</u> 1607 bmr<u>F</u> 1426   hgt 74 bmr<u>M</u> 1632 bmr<u>F</u> 1435
hgt 76 bmr<u>M</u> 1658 bmr<u>F</u> 1444   hgt 78 bmr<u>M</u> 1683 bmr<u>F</u> 1453

weight 160

hgt 60 bmr<u>M</u> 1517 bmr<u>F</u> 1415   hgt 62 bmr<u>M</u> 1542 bmr<u>F</u> 1424
hgt 64 bmr<u>M</u> 1567 bmr<u>F</u> 1433   hgt 66 bmr<u>M</u> 1593 bmr<u>F</u> 1442
hgt 68 bmr<u>M</u> 1618 bmr<u>F</u> 1451   hgt 70 bmr<u>M</u> 1644 bmr<u>F</u> 1461
hgt 72 bmr<u>M</u> 1669 bmr<u>F</u> 1470   hgt 74 bmr<u>M</u> 1694 bmr<u>F</u> 1479
hgt 76 bmr<u>M</u> 1720 bmr<u>F</u> 1488   hgt 78 bmr<u>M</u> 1745 bmr<u>F</u> 1497

weight 170

hgt 60 bmr<u>M</u> 1579 bmr<u>F</u> 1458   hgt 62 bmr<u>M</u> 1604 bmr<u>F</u> 1468
hgt 64 bmr<u>M</u> 1630 bmr<u>F</u> 1477   hgt 66 bmr<u>M</u> 1655 bmr<u>F</u> 1486
hgt 68 bmr<u>M</u> 1680 bmr<u>F</u> 1495   hgt 70 bmr<u>M</u> 1706 bmr<u>F</u> 1504
hgt 72 bmr<u>M</u> 1731 bmr<u>F</u> 1513   hgt 74 bmr<u>M</u> 1757 bmr<u>F</u> 1522
hgt 76 bmr<u>M</u> 1782 bmr<u>F</u> 1532   hgt 78 bmr<u>M</u> 1807 bmr<u>F</u> 1541

weight 180

hgt 60 bmr<u>M</u> 1641 bmr<u>F</u> 1502   hgt 62 bmr<u>M</u> 1666 bmr<u>F</u> 1511
hgt 64 bmr<u>M</u> 1692 bmr<u>F</u> 1520   hgt 66 bmr<u>M</u> 1717 bmr<u>F</u> 1529
hgt 68 bmr<u>M</u> 1743 bmr<u>F</u> 1539   hgt 70 bmr<u>M</u> 1768 bmr<u>F</u> 1548
hgt 72 bmr<u>M</u> 1793 bmr<u>F</u> 1557   hgt 74 bmr<u>M</u> 1819 bmr<u>F</u> 1566
hgt 76 bmr<u>M</u> 1844 bmr<u>F</u> 1575   hgt 78 bmr<u>M</u> 1870 bmr<u>F</u> 1584

weight 190

hgt 60 bmr<u>M</u> 1703 bmr<u>F</u> 1546   hgt 62 bmr<u>M</u> 1729 bmr<u>F</u> 1555
hgt 64 bmr<u>M</u> 1754 bmr<u>F</u> 1564   hgt 66 bmr<u>M</u> 1779 bmr<u>F</u> 1573
hgt 68 bmr<u>M</u> 1805 bmr<u>F</u> 1582   hgt 70 bmr<u>M</u> 1830 bmr<u>F</u> 1591
hgt 72 bmr<u>M</u> 1856 bmr<u>F</u> 1600   hgt 74 bmr<u>M</u> 1881 bmr<u>F</u> 1610
hgt 76 bmr<u>M</u> 1906 bmr<u>F</u> 1619   hgt 78 bmr<u>M</u> 1932 bmr<u>F</u> 1628

weight 200

hgt 60 bmr<u>M</u> 1765 bmr<u>F</u> 1589   hgt 62 bmr<u>M</u> 1791 bmr<u>F</u> 1598
hgt 64 bmr<u>M</u> 1816 bmr<u>F</u> 1607   hgt 66 bmr<u>M</u> 1842 bmr<u>F</u> 1617
hgt 68 bmr<u>M</u> 1867 bmr<u>F</u> 1626   hgt 70 bmr<u>M</u> 1892 bmr<u>F</u> 1635
hgt 72 bmr<u>M</u> 1918 bmr<u>F</u> 1644   hgt 74 bmr<u>M</u> 1943 bmr<u>F</u> 1653
hgt 76 bmr<u>M</u> 1969 bmr<u>F</u> 1662   hgt 78 bmr<u>M</u> 1994 bmr<u>F</u> 1671

weight 210

hgt 60 bmr<u>M</u> 1828 bmr<u>F</u> 1633   hgt 62 bmr<u>M</u> 1853 bmr<u>F</u> 1642
hgt 64 bmr<u>M</u> 1878 bmr<u>F</u> 1651   hgt 66 bmr<u>M</u> 1904 bmr<u>F</u> 1660
hgt 68 bmr<u>M</u> 1929 bmr<u>F</u> 1669   hgt 70 bmr<u>M</u> 1955 bmr<u>F</u> 1679
hgt 72 bmr<u>M</u> 1980 bmr<u>F</u> 1688   hgt 74 bmr<u>M</u> 2005 bmr<u>F</u> 1697
hgt 76 bmr<u>M</u> 2031 bmr<u>F</u> 1706   hgt 78 bmr<u>M</u> 2056 bmr<u>F</u> 1715

weight 220

hgt 60 bmr<u>M</u> 1890 bmr<u>F</u> 1676   hgt 62 bmr<u>M</u> 1915 bmr<u>F</u> 1686
hgt 64 bmr<u>M</u> 1941 bmr<u>F</u> 1695   hgt 66 bmr<u>M</u> 1966 bmr<u>F</u> 1704
hgt 68 bmr<u>M</u> 1991 bmr<u>F</u> 1713   hgt 70 bmr<u>M</u> 2017 bmr<u>F</u> 1722
hgt 72 bmr<u>M</u> 2042 bmr<u>F</u> 1731   hgt 74 bmr<u>M</u> 2068 bmr<u>F</u> 1740
hgt 76 bmr<u>M</u> 2093 bmr<u>F</u> 1750   hgt 78 bmr<u>M</u> 2118 bmr<u>F</u> 1759

weight 230

hgt 60 bmr<u>M</u> 1952 bmr<u>F</u> 1720   hgt 62 hmr<u>M</u> 1977 hmr<u>F</u> 1729
hgt 64 bmr<u>M</u> 2003 bmr<u>F</u> 1738   hgt 66 bmr<u>M</u> 2028 bmr<u>F</u> 1747
hgt 68 bmr<u>M</u> 2054 bmr<u>F</u> 1757   hgt 70 bmr<u>M</u> 2079 bmr<u>F</u> 1766
hgt 72 bmr<u>M</u> 2104 bmr<u>F</u> 1775   hgt 74 bmr<u>M</u> 2130 bmr<u>F</u> 1784
hgt 76 bmr<u>M</u> 2155 bmr<u>F</u> 1793   hgt 78 bmr<u>M</u> 2181 bmr<u>F</u> 1802

weight 240

hgt 60 bmr<u>M</u> 2014 bmr<u>F</u> 1764 hgt 62 bmr<u>M</u> 2040 bmr<u>F</u> 1773
hgt 64 bmr<u>M</u> 2065 bmr<u>F</u> 1782 hgt 66 bmr<u>M</u> 2090 bmr<u>F</u> 1791
hgt 68 bmr<u>M</u> 2116 bmr<u>F</u> 1800 hgt 70 bmr<u>M</u> 2141 bmr<u>F</u> 1809
hgt 72 bmr<u>M</u> 2167 bmr<u>F</u> 1818 hgt 74 bmr<u>M</u> 2192 bmr<u>F</u> 1828
hgt 76 bmr<u>M</u> 2217 bmr<u>F</u> 1837 hgt 78 bmr<u>M</u> 2243 bmr<u>F</u> 1846

weight 250

hgt 60 bmr<u>M</u> 2076 bmr<u>F</u> 1807 hgt 62 bmr<u>M</u> 2102 bmr<u>F</u> 1816
hgt 64 bmr<u>M</u> 2127 bmr<u>F</u> 1825 hgt 66 bmr<u>M</u> 2153 bmr<u>F</u> 1835
hgt 68 bmr<u>M</u> 2178 bmr<u>F</u> 1844 hgt 70 bmr<u>M</u> 2203 bmr<u>F</u> 1853
hgt 72 bmr<u>M</u> 2229 bmr<u>F</u> 1862 hgt 74 bmr<u>M</u> 2254 bmr<u>F</u> 1871
hgt 76 bmr<u>M</u> 2280 bmr<u>F</u> 1880 hgt 78 bmr<u>M</u> 2305 bmr<u>F</u> 1889

weight 260

hgt 60 bmr<u>M</u> 2139 bmr<u>F</u> 1851 hgt 62 bmr<u>M</u> 2164 bmr<u>F</u> 1860
hgt 64 bmr<u>M</u> 2189 bmr<u>F</u> 1869 hgt 66 bmr<u>M</u> 2215 bmr<u>F</u> 1878
hgt 68 bmr<u>M</u> 2240 bmr<u>F</u> 1887 hgt 70 bmr<u>M</u> 2266 bmr<u>F</u> 1897
hgt 72 bmr<u>M</u> 2291 bmr<u>F</u> 1906 hgt 74 bmr<u>M</u> 2316 bmr<u>F</u> 1915
hgt 76 bmr<u>M</u> 2342 bmr<u>F</u> 1924 hgt 78 bmr<u>M</u> 2367 bmr<u>F</u> 1933

weight 270

hgt 60 bmr<u>M</u> 2201 bmr<u>F</u> 1894 hgt 62 bmr<u>M</u> 2226 bmr<u>F</u> 1904
hgt 64 bmr<u>M</u> 2252 bmr<u>F</u> 1913 hgt 66 bmr<u>M</u> 2277 bmr<u>F</u> 1922
hgt 68 bmr<u>M</u> 2302 bmr<u>F</u> 1931 hgt 70 bmr<u>M</u> 2328 bmr<u>F</u> 1940
hgt 72 bmr<u>M</u> 2353 bmr<u>F</u> 1949 hgt 74 bmr<u>M</u> 2379 bmr<u>F</u> 1958
hgt 76 bmr<u>M</u> 2404 bmr<u>F</u> 1968 hgt 78 bmr<u>M</u> 2429 bmr<u>F</u> 1977

weight 280

hgt 60 bmr<u>M</u> 2263 bmr<u>F</u> 1938 hgt 62 bmr<u>M</u> 2288 bmr<u>F</u> 1947
hgt 64 bmr<u>M</u> 2314 bmr<u>F</u> 1956 hgt 66 bmr<u>M</u> 2339 bmr<u>F</u> 1965
hgt 68 bmr<u>M</u> 2365 bmr<u>F</u> 1975 hgt 70 bmr<u>M</u> 2390 bmr<u>F</u> 1984
hgt 72 bmr<u>M</u> 2415 bmr<u>F</u> 1993 hgt 74 bmr<u>M</u> 2441 bmr<u>F</u> 2002
hgt 76 bmr<u>M</u> 2466 bmr<u>F</u> 2011 hgt 78 bmr<u>M</u> 2492 bmr<u>F</u> 2020

weight 290

hgt 60 bmr<u>M</u> 2325 bmr<u>F</u> 1982 hgt 62 bmr<u>M</u> 2351 bmr<u>F</u> 1991
hgt 64 bmr<u>M</u> 2376 bmr<u>F</u> 2000 hgt 66 bmr<u>M</u> 2401 bmr<u>F</u> 2009
hgt 68 bmr<u>M</u> 2427 bmr<u>F</u> 2018 hgt 70 bmr<u>M</u> 2452 bmr<u>F</u> 2027
hgt 72 bmr<u>M</u> 2478 bmr<u>F</u> 2036 hgt 74 bmr<u>M</u> 2503 bmr<u>F</u> 2046
hgt 76 bmr<u>M</u> 2528 bmr<u>F</u> 2055 hgt 78 bmr<u>M</u> 2554 bmr<u>F</u> 2064

weight 300

hgt 60 bmr<u>M</u> 2387 bmr<u>F</u> 2025 hgt 62 bmr<u>M</u> 2413 bmr<u>F</u> 2034
hgt 64 bmr<u>M</u> 2438 bmr<u>F</u> 2043 hgt 66 bmr<u>M</u> 2464 bmr<u>F</u> 2053
hgt 68 bmr<u>M</u> 2489 bmr<u>F</u> 2062 hgt 70 bmr<u>M</u> 2514 bmr<u>F</u> 2071
hgt 72 bmr<u>M</u> 2540 bmr<u>F</u> 2080 hgt 74 bmr<u>M</u> 2565 bmr<u>F</u> 2089
hgt 76 bmr<u>M</u> 2591 bmr<u>F</u> 2098 hgt 78 bmr<u>M</u> 2616 bmr<u>F</u> 2107

Age 50

weight 110

hgt 60 bmr<u>M</u> 1172 bmr<u>F</u> 1173 hgt 62 bmr<u>M</u> 1197 bmr<u>F</u> 1182
hgt 64 bmr<u>M</u> 1222 bmr<u>F</u> 1192 hgt 66 bmr<u>M</u> 1248 bmr<u>F</u> 1201
hgt 68 bmr<u>M</u> 1273 bmr<u>F</u> 1210 hgt 70 bmr<u>M</u> 1299 bmr<u>F</u> 1219
hgt 72 bmr<u>M</u> 1324 bmr<u>F</u> 1228 hgt 74 bmr<u>M</u> 1349 bmr<u>F</u> 1237
hgt 76 bmr<u>M</u> 1375 bmr<u>F</u> 1246 hgt 78 bmr<u>M</u> 1400 bmr<u>F</u> 1256

weight 120

hgt 60 bmr<u>M</u> 1234 bmr<u>F</u> 1217 hgt 62 bmr<u>M</u> 1259 bmr<u>F</u> 1226
hgt 64 bmr<u>M</u> 1285 bmr<u>F</u> 1235 hgt 66 bmr<u>M</u> 1310 bmr<u>F</u> 1244
hgt 68 bmr<u>M</u> 1335 bmr<u>F</u> 1253 hgt 70 bmr<u>M</u> 1361 bmr<u>F</u> 1263
hgt 72 bmr<u>M</u> 1386 bmr<u>F</u> 1272 hgt 74 bmr<u>M</u> 1412 bmr<u>F</u> 1281
hgt 76 bmr<u>M</u> 1437 bmr<u>F</u> 1290 hgt 78 bmr<u>M</u> 1462 bmr<u>F</u> 1299

weight 130

hgt 60 bmr<u>M</u> 1296 bmr<u>F</u> 1261 hgt 62 bmr<u>M</u> 1321 bmr<u>F</u> 1270
hgt 64 bmr<u>M</u> 1347 bmr<u>F</u> 1279 hgt 66 bmr<u>M</u> 1372 bmr<u>F</u> 1288
hgt 68 bmr<u>M</u> 1398 bmr<u>F</u> 1297 hgt 70 bmr<u>M</u> 1423 bmr<u>F</u> 1306
hgt 72 bmr<u>M</u> 1448 bmr<u>F</u> 1315 hgt 74 bmr<u>M</u> 1474 bmr<u>F</u> 1324
hgt 76 bmr<u>M</u> 1499 bmr<u>F</u> 1334 hgt 78 bmr<u>M</u> 1525 bmr<u>F</u> 1343

weight 140

hgt 60 bmr<u>M</u> 1358 bmr<u>F</u> 1304 hgt 62 bmr<u>M</u> 1384 bmr<u>F</u> 1313
hgt 64 bmr<u>M</u> 1409 bmr<u>F</u> 1322 hgt 66 bmr<u>M</u> 1434 bmr<u>F</u> 1332
hgt 68 bmr<u>M</u> 1460 bmr<u>F</u> 1341 hgt 70 bmr<u>M</u> 1485 bmr<u>F</u> 1350
hgt 72 bmr<u>M</u> 1511 bmr<u>F</u> 1359 hgt 74 bmr<u>M</u> 1536 bmr<u>F</u> 1368
hgt 76 bmr<u>M</u> 1561 bmr<u>F</u> 1377 hgt 78 bmr<u>M</u> 1587 bmr<u>F</u> 1386

weight 150

hgt 60 bmr<u>M</u> 1420 bmr<u>F</u> 1348 hgt 62 bmr<u>M</u> 1446 bmr<u>F</u> 1357
hgt 64 bmr<u>M</u> 1471 bmr<u>F</u> 1366 hgt 66 bmr<u>M</u> 1497 bmr<u>F</u> 1375
hgt 68 bmr<u>M</u> 1522 bmr<u>F</u> 1384 hgt 70 bmr<u>M</u> 1547 bmr<u>F</u> 1393
hgt 72 bmr<u>M</u> 1573 bmr<u>F</u> 1403 hgt 74 bmr<u>M</u> 1598 bmr<u>F</u> 1412
hgt 76 bmr<u>M</u> 1624 bmr<u>F</u> 1421 hgt 78 bmr<u>M</u> 1649 bmr<u>F</u> 1430

weight 160
hgt 60 bmr<u>M</u> 1483 bmr<u>F</u> 1391 hgt 62 bmr<u>M</u> 1508 bmr<u>F</u> 1400
hgt 64 bmr<u>M</u> 1533 bmr<u>F</u> 1410 hgt 66 bmr<u>M</u> 1559 bmr<u>F</u> 1419
hgt 68 bmr<u>M</u> 1584 bmr<u>F</u> 1428 hgt 70 bmr<u>M</u> 1610 bmr<u>F</u> 1437
hgt 72 bmr<u>M</u> 1635 bmr<u>F</u> 1446 hgt 74 bmr<u>M</u> 1660 bmr<u>F</u> 1455
hgt 76 bmr<u>M</u> 1686 bmr<u>F</u> 1464 hgt 78 bmr<u>M</u> 1711 bmr<u>F</u> 1474

weight 170
hgt 60 bmr<u>M</u> 1545 bmr<u>F</u> 1435 hgt 62 bmr<u>M</u> 1570 bmr<u>F</u> 1444
hgt 64 bmr<u>M</u> 1596 bmr<u>F</u> 1453 hgt 66 bmr<u>M</u> 1621 bmr<u>F</u> 1462
hgt 68 bmr<u>M</u> 1646 bmr<u>F</u> 1471 hgt 70 bmr<u>M</u> 1672 bmr<u>F</u> 1481
hgt 72 bmr<u>M</u> 1697 bmr<u>F</u> 1490 hgt 74 bmr<u>M</u> 1723 bmr<u>F</u> 1499
hgt 76 bmr<u>M</u> 1748 bmr<u>F</u> 1508 hgt 78 bmr<u>M</u> 1773 bmr<u>F</u> 1517

weight 180
hgt 60 bmr<u>M</u> 1607 bmr<u>F</u> 1479 hgt 62 bmr<u>M</u> 1632 bmr<u>F</u> 1488
hgt 64 bmr<u>M</u> 1658 bmr<u>F</u> 1497 hgt 66 bmr<u>M</u> 1683 bmr<u>F</u> 1506
hgt 68 bmr<u>M</u> 1709 bmr<u>F</u> 1515 hgt 70 bmr<u>M</u> 1734 bmr<u>F</u> 1524
hgt 72 bmr<u>M</u> 1759 bmr<u>F</u> 1533 hgt 74 bmr<u>M</u> 1785 bmr<u>F</u> 1542
hgt 76 bmr<u>M</u> 1810 bmr<u>F</u> 1552 hgt 78 bmr<u>M</u> 1836 bmr<u>F</u> 1561

weight 190
hgt 60 bmr<u>M</u> 1669 bmr<u>F</u> 1522 hgt 62 bmr<u>M</u> 1695 bmr<u>F</u> 1531
hgt 64 bmr<u>M</u> 1720 bmr<u>F</u> 1540 hgt 66 bmr<u>M</u> 1745 bmr<u>F</u> 1550
hgt 68 bmr<u>M</u> 1771 bmr<u>F</u> 1559 hgt 70 bmr<u>M</u> 1796 bmr<u>F</u> 1568
hgt 72 bmr<u>M</u> 1822 bmr<u>F</u> 1577 hgt 74 bmr<u>M</u> 1847 bmr<u>F</u> 1586
hgt 76 bmr<u>M</u> 1872 bmr<u>F</u> 1595 hgt 78 bmr<u>M</u> 1898 bmr<u>F</u> 1604

weight 200
hgt 60 bmr<u>M</u> 1731 bmr<u>F</u> 1566 hgt 62 bmr<u>M</u> 1757 bmr<u>F</u> 1575
hgt 64 bmr<u>M</u> 1782 bmr<u>F</u> 1584 hgt 66 bmr<u>M</u> 1808 bmr<u>F</u> 1593
hgt 68 bmr<u>M</u> 1833 bmr<u>F</u> 1602 hgt 70 bmr<u>M</u> 1858 bmr<u>F</u> 1611
hgt 72 bmr<u>M</u> 1884 bmr<u>F</u> 1621 hgt 74 bmr<u>M</u> 1909 bmr<u>F</u> 1630
hgt 76 bmr<u>M</u> 1935 bmr<u>F</u> 1639 hgt 78 bmr<u>M</u> 1960 bmr<u>F</u> 1648

weight 210
hgt 60 bmr<u>M</u> 1794 bmr<u>F</u> 1609 hgt 62 bmr<u>M</u> 1819 bmr<u>F</u> 1618
hgt 64 bmr<u>M</u> 1844 bmr<u>F</u> 1628 hgt 66 bmr<u>M</u> 1870 bmr<u>F</u> 1637
hgt 68 bmr<u>M</u> 1895 bmr<u>F</u> 1646 hgt 70 bmr<u>M</u> 1921 bmr<u>F</u> 1655
hgt 72 bmr<u>M</u> 1946 bmr<u>F</u> 1664 hgt 74 bmr<u>M</u> 1971 bmr<u>F</u> 1673
hgt 76 bmr<u>M</u> 1997 bmr<u>F</u> 1682 hgt 78 bmr<u>M</u> 2022 bmr<u>F</u> 1692

weight 220

hgt 60 bmr<u>M</u> 1856 bmr<u>F</u> 1653   hgt 62 bmr<u>M</u> 1881 bmr<u>F</u> 1662
hgt 64 bmr<u>M</u> 1907 bmr<u>F</u> 1671   hgt 66 bmr<u>M</u> 1932 bmr<u>F</u> 1680
hgt 68 bmr<u>M</u> 1957 bmr<u>F</u> 1689   hgt 70 bmr<u>M</u> 1983 bmr<u>F</u> 1699
hgt 72 bmr<u>M</u> 2008 bmr<u>F</u> 1708   hgt 74 bmr<u>M</u> 2034 bmr<u>F</u> 1717
hgt 76 bmr<u>M</u> 2059 bmr<u>F</u> 1726   hgt 78 bmr<u>M</u> 2084 bmr<u>F</u> 1735

weight 230

hgt 60 bmr<u>M</u> 1918 bmr<u>F</u> 1697   hgt 62 bmr<u>M</u> 1943 bmr<u>F</u> 1706
hgt 64 bmr<u>M</u> 1969 bmr<u>F</u> 1715   hgt 66 bmr<u>M</u> 1994 bmr<u>F</u> 1724
hgt 68 bmr<u>M</u> 2020 bmr<u>F</u> 1733   hgt 70 bmr<u>M</u> 2045 bmr<u>F</u> 1742
hgt 72 bmr<u>M</u> 2070 bmr<u>F</u> 1751   hgt 74 bmr<u>M</u> 2096 bmr<u>F</u> 1760
hgt 76 bmr<u>M</u> 2121 bmr<u>F</u> 1770   hgt 78 bmr<u>M</u> 2147 bmr<u>F</u> 1779

weight 240

hgt 60 bmr<u>M</u> 1980 bmr<u>F</u> 1740   hgt 62 bmr<u>M</u> 2006 bmr<u>F</u> 1749
hgt 64 bmr<u>M</u> 2031 bmr<u>F</u> 1758   hgt 66 bmr<u>M</u> 2056 bmr<u>F</u> 1768
hgt 68 bmr<u>M</u> 2082 bmr<u>F</u> 1777   hgt 70 bmr<u>M</u> 2107 bmr<u>F</u> 1786
hgt 72 bmr<u>M</u> 2133 bmr<u>F</u> 1795   hgt 74 bmr<u>M</u> 2158 bmr<u>F</u> 1804
hgt 76 bmr<u>M</u> 2183 bmr<u>F</u> 1813   hgt 78 bmr<u>M</u> 2209 bmr<u>F</u> 1822

weight 250

hgt 60 bmr<u>M</u> 2042 bmr<u>F</u> 1784   hgt 62 bmr<u>M</u> 2068 bmr<u>F</u> 1793
hgt 64 bmr<u>M</u> 2093 bmr<u>F</u> 1802   hgt 66 bmr<u>M</u> 2119 bmr<u>F</u> 1811
hgt 68 bmr<u>M</u> 2144 bmr<u>F</u> 1820   hgt 70 bmr<u>M</u> 2169 bmr<u>F</u> 1829
hgt 72 bmr<u>M</u> 2195 bmr<u>F</u> 1839   hgt 74 bmr<u>M</u> 2220 bmr<u>F</u> 1848
hgt 76 bmr<u>M</u> 2246 bmr<u>F</u> 1857   hgt 78 bmr<u>M</u> 2271 bmr<u>F</u> 1866

weight 260

hgt 60 bmr<u>M</u> 2105 bmr<u>F</u> 1827   hgt 62 bmr<u>M</u> 2130 bmr<u>F</u> 1836
hgt 64 bmr<u>M</u> 2155 bmr<u>F</u> 1846   hgt 66 bmr<u>M</u> 2181 bmr<u>F</u> 1855
hgt 68 bmr<u>M</u> 2206 bmr<u>F</u> 1864   hgt 70 bmr<u>M</u> 2232 bmr<u>F</u> 1873
hgt 72 bmr<u>M</u> 2257 bmr<u>F</u> 1882   hgt 74 bmr<u>M</u> 2282 bmr<u>F</u> 1891
hgt 76 bmr<u>M</u> 2308 bmr<u>F</u> 1900   hgt 78 bmr<u>M</u> 2333 bmr<u>F</u> 1910

weight 270

hgt 60 bmr<u>M</u> 2167 bmr<u>F</u> 1871   hgt 62 bmr<u>M</u> 2192 bmr<u>F</u> 1880
hgt 64 bmr<u>M</u> 2218 bmr<u>F</u> 1889   hgt 66 bmr<u>M</u> 2243 bmr<u>F</u> 1898
hgt 68 bmr<u>M</u> 2268 bmr<u>F</u> 1907   hgt 70 bmr<u>M</u> 2294 bmr<u>F</u> 1917
hgt 72 bmr<u>M</u> 2319 bmr<u>F</u> 1926   hgt 74 bmr<u>M</u> 2345 bmr<u>F</u> 1935
hgt 76 bmr<u>M</u> 2370 bmr<u>F</u> 1944   hgt 78 bmr<u>M</u> 2395 bmr<u>F</u> 1953

weight 280
hgt 60 bmr<u>M</u> 2229 bmr<u>F</u> 1915 hgt 62 bmr<u>M</u> 2254 bmr<u>F</u> 1924
hgt 64 bmr<u>M</u> 2280 bmr<u>F</u> 1933 hgt 66 bmr<u>M</u> 2305 bmr<u>F</u> 1942
hgt 68 bmr<u>M</u> 2331 bmr<u>F</u> 1951 hgt 70 bmr<u>M</u> 2356 bmr<u>F</u> 1960
hgt 72 bmr<u>M</u> 2381 bmr<u>F</u> 1969 hgt 74 bmr<u>M</u> 2407 bmr<u>F</u> 1978
hgt 76 bmr<u>M</u> 2432 bmr<u>F</u> 1988 hgt 78 bmr<u>M</u> 2458 bmr<u>F</u> 1997

weight 290
hgt 60 bmr<u>M</u> 2291 bmr<u>F</u> 1958 hgt 62 bmr<u>M</u> 2317 bmr<u>F</u> 1967
hgt 64 bmr<u>M</u> 2342 bmr<u>F</u> 1976 hgt 66 bmr<u>M</u> 2367 bmr<u>F</u> 1986
hgt 68 bmr<u>M</u> 2393 bmr<u>F</u> 1995 hgt 70 bmr<u>M</u> 2418 bmr<u>F</u> 2004
hgt 72 bmr<u>M</u> 2444 bmr<u>F</u> 2013 hgt 74 bmr<u>M</u> 2469 bmr<u>F</u> 2022
hgt 76 bmr<u>M</u> 2494 bmr<u>F</u> 2031 hgt 78 bmr<u>M</u> 2520 bmr<u>F</u> 2040

weight 300
hgt 60 bmr<u>M</u> 2353 bmr<u>F</u> 2002 hgt 62 bmr<u>M</u> 2379 bmr<u>F</u> 2011
hgt 64 bmr<u>M</u> 2404 bmr<u>F</u> 2020 hgt 66 bmr<u>M</u> 2430 bmr<u>F</u> 2029
hgt 68 bmr<u>M</u> 2455 bmr<u>F</u> 2038 hgt 70 bmr<u>M</u> 2480 bmr<u>F</u> 2047
hgt 72 bmr<u>M</u> 2506 bmr<u>F</u> 2057 hgt 74 bmr<u>M</u> 2531 bmr<u>F</u> 2066
hgt 76 bmr<u>M</u> 2557 bmr<u>F</u> 2075 hgt 78 bmr<u>M</u> 2582 bmr<u>F</u> 2084

Age 55

weight 110
hgt 60 bmr<u>M</u> 1138 bmr<u>F</u> 1150 hgt 62 bmr<u>M</u> 1163 bmr<u>F</u> 1159
hgt 64 bmr<u>M</u> 1188 bmr<u>F</u> 1168 hgt 66 bmr<u>M</u> 1214 bmr<u>F</u> 1177
hgt 68 bmr<u>M</u> 1239 bmr<u>F</u> 1186 hgt 70 bmr<u>M</u> 1265 bmr<u>F</u> 1196
hgt 72 bmr<u>M</u> 1290 bmr<u>F</u> 1205 hgt 74 bmr<u>M</u> 1315 bmr<u>F</u> 1214
hgt 76 bmr<u>M</u> 1341 bmr<u>F</u> 1223 hgt 78 bmr<u>M</u> 1366 bmr<u>F</u> 1232

weight 120
hgt 60 bmr<u>M</u> 1200 bmr<u>F</u> 1193 hgt 62 bmr<u>M</u> 1225 bmr<u>F</u> 1203
hgt 64 bmr<u>M</u> 1251 bmr<u>F</u> 1212 hgt 66 bmr<u>M</u> 1276 bmr<u>F</u> 1221
hgt 68 bmr<u>M</u> 1301 bmr<u>F</u> 1230 hgt 70 bmr<u>M</u> 1327 bmr<u>F</u> 1239
hgt 72 bmr<u>M</u> 1352 bmr<u>F</u> 1248 hgt 74 bmr<u>M</u> 1378 bmr<u>F</u> 1257
hgt 76 bmr<u>M</u> 1403 bmr<u>F</u> 1267 hgt 78 bmr<u>M</u> 1428 bmr<u>F</u> 1276

weight 130
hgt 60 bmr<u>M</u> 1262 bmr<u>F</u> 1237 hgt 62 bmr<u>M</u> 1287 bmr<u>F</u> 1246
hgt 64 bmr<u>M</u> 1313 bmr<u>F</u> 1255 hgt 66 bmr<u>M</u> 1338 bmr<u>F</u> 1264
hgt 68 bmr<u>M</u> 1364 bmr<u>F</u> 1274 hgt 70 bmr<u>M</u> 1389 bmr<u>F</u> 1283
hgt 72 bmr<u>M</u> 1414 bmr<u>F</u> 1292 hgt 74 bmr<u>M</u> 1440 bmr<u>F</u> 1301
hgt 76 bmr<u>M</u> 1465 bmr<u>F</u> 1310 hgt 78 bmr<u>M</u> 1491 bmr<u>F</u> 1319

<u>weight</u> 140

hgt 60 bmr<u>M</u> 1324 bmr<u>F</u> 1281   hgt 62 bmr<u>M</u> 1350 bmr<u>F</u> 1290
hgt 64 bmr<u>M</u> 1375 bmr<u>F</u> 1299   hgt 66 bmr<u>M</u> 1400 bmr<u>F</u> 1308
hgt 68 bmr<u>M</u> 1426 bmr<u>F</u> 1317   hgt 70 bmr<u>M</u> 1451 bmr<u>F</u> 1326
hgt 72 bmr<u>M</u> 1477 bmr<u>F</u> 1335   hgt 74 bmr<u>M</u> 1502 bmr<u>F</u> 1345
hgt 76 bmr<u>M</u> 1527 bmr<u>F</u> 1354   hgt 78 bmr<u>M</u> 1553 bmr<u>F</u> 1363

<u>weight</u> 150

hgt 60 bmr<u>M</u> 1386 bmr<u>F</u> 1324   hgt 62 bmr<u>M</u> 1412 bmr<u>F</u> 1333
hgt 64 bmr<u>M</u> 1437 bmr<u>F</u> 1342   hgt 66 bmr<u>M</u> 1463 bmr<u>F</u> 1352
hgt 68 bmr<u>M</u> 1488 bmr<u>F</u> 1361   hgt 70 bmr<u>M</u> 1513 bmr<u>F</u> 1370
hgt 72 bmr<u>M</u> 1539 bmr<u>F</u> 1379   hgt 74 bmr<u>M</u> 1564 bmr<u>F</u> 1388
hgt 76 bmr<u>M</u> 1590 bmr<u>F</u> 1397   hgt 78 bmr<u>M</u> 1615 bmr<u>F</u> 1406

<u>weight</u> 160

hgt 60 bmr<u>M</u> 1449 bmr<u>F</u> 1368   hgt 62 bmr<u>M</u> 1474 bmr<u>F</u> 1377
hgt 64 bmr<u>M</u> 1499 bmr<u>F</u> 1386   hgt 66 bmr<u>M</u> 1525 bmr<u>F</u> 1395
hgt 68 bmr<u>M</u> 1550 bmr<u>F</u> 1404   hgt 70 bmr<u>M</u> 1576 bmr<u>F</u> 1414
hgt 72 bmr<u>M</u> 1601 bmr<u>F</u> 1423   hgt 74 bmr<u>M</u> 1626 bmr<u>F</u> 1432
hgt 76 bmr<u>M</u> 1652 bmr<u>F</u> 1441   hgt 78 bmr<u>M</u> 1677 bmr<u>F</u> 1450

<u>weight</u> 170

hgt 60 bmr<u>M</u> 1511 bmr<u>F</u> 1411   hgt 62 bmr<u>M</u> 1536 bmr<u>F</u> 1421
hgt 64 bmr<u>M</u> 1562 bmr<u>F</u> 1430   hgt 66 bmr<u>M</u> 1587 bmr<u>F</u> 1439
hgt 68 bmr<u>M</u> 1612 bmr<u>F</u> 1448   hgt 70 bmr<u>M</u> 1638 bmr<u>F</u> 1457
hgt 72 bmr<u>M</u> 1663 bmr<u>F</u> 1466   hgt 74 bmr<u>M</u> 1689 bmr<u>F</u> 1475
hgt 76 bmr<u>M</u> 1714 bmr<u>F</u> 1485   hgt 78 bmr<u>M</u> 1739 bmr<u>F</u> 1494

<u>weight</u> 180

hgt 60 bmr<u>M</u> 1573 bmr<u>F</u> 1455   hgt 62 bmr<u>M</u> 1598 bmr<u>F</u> 1464
hgt 64 bmr<u>M</u> 1624 bmr<u>F</u> 1473   hgt 66 bmr<u>M</u> 1649 bmr<u>F</u> 1482
hgt 68 bmr<u>M</u> 1675 bmr<u>F</u> 1492   hgt 70 bmr<u>M</u> 1700 bmr<u>F</u> 1501
hgt 72 bmr<u>M</u> 1725 bmr<u>F</u> 1510   hgt 74 bmr<u>M</u> 1751 bmr<u>F</u> 1519
hgt 76 bmr<u>M</u> 1776 bmr<u>F</u> 1528   hgt 78 bmr<u>M</u> 1802 bmr<u>F</u> 1537

<u>weight</u> 190

hgt 60 bmr<u>M</u> 1635 bmr<u>F</u> 1499   hgt 62 bmr<u>M</u> 1661 bmr<u>F</u> 1508
hgt 64 bmr<u>M</u> 1686 bmr<u>F</u> 1517   hgt 66 bmr<u>M</u> 1711 bmr<u>F</u> 1526
hgt 68 bmr<u>M</u> 1737 bmr<u>F</u> 1535   hgt 70 bmr<u>M</u> 1762 bmr<u>F</u> 1544
hgt 72 bmr<u>M</u> 1788 bmr<u>F</u> 1553   hgt 74 bmr<u>M</u> 1813 bmr<u>F</u> 1563
hgt 76 bmr<u>M</u> 1838 bmr<u>F</u> 1572   hgt 78 bmr<u>M</u> 1864 bmr<u>F</u> 1581

weight 200

hgt 60 bmr<u>M</u> 1697 bmr<u>F</u> 1542 hgt 62 bmr<u>M</u> 1723 bmr<u>F</u> 1551
hgt 64 bmr<u>M</u> 1748 bmr<u>F</u> 1560 hgt 66 bmr<u>M</u> 1774 bmr<u>F</u> 1570
hgt 68 bmr<u>M</u> 1799 bmr<u>F</u> 1579 hgt 70 bmr<u>M</u> 1824 bmr<u>F</u> 1588
hgt 72 bmr<u>M</u> 1850 bmr<u>F</u> 1597 hgt 74 bmr<u>M</u> 1875 bmr<u>F</u> 1606
hgt 76 bmr<u>M</u> 1901 bmr<u>F</u> 1615 hgt 78 bmr<u>M</u> 1926 bmr<u>F</u> 1624

weight 210

hgt 60 bmr<u>M</u> 1760 bmr<u>F</u> 1586 hgt 62 bmr<u>M</u> 1785 bmr<u>F</u> 1595
hgt 64 bmr<u>M</u> 1810 bmr<u>F</u> 1604 hgt 66 bmr<u>M</u> 1836 bmr<u>F</u> 1613
hgt 68 bmr<u>M</u> 1861 bmr<u>F</u> 1622 hgt 70 bmr<u>M</u> 1887 bmr<u>F</u> 1632
hgt 72 bmr<u>M</u> 1912 bmr<u>F</u> 1641 hgt 74 bmr<u>M</u> 1937 bmr<u>F</u> 1650
hgt 76 bmr<u>M</u> 1963 bmr<u>F</u> 1659 hgt 78 bmr<u>M</u> 1988 bmr<u>F</u> 1668

weight 220

hgt 60 bmr<u>M</u> 1822 bmr<u>F</u> 1629 hgt 62 bmr<u>M</u> 1847 bmr<u>F</u> 1639
hgt 64 bmr<u>M</u> 1873 bmr<u>F</u> 1648 hgt 66 bmr<u>M</u> 1898 bmr<u>F</u> 1657
hgt 68 bmr<u>M</u> 1923 bmr<u>F</u> 1666 hgt 70 bmr<u>M</u> 1949 bmr<u>F</u> 1675
hgt 72 bmr<u>M</u> 1974 bmr<u>F</u> 1684 hgt 74 bmr<u>M</u> 2000 bmr<u>F</u> 1693
hgt 76 bmr<u>M</u> 2025 bmr<u>F</u> 1703 hgt 78 bmr<u>M</u> 2050 bmr<u>F</u> 1712

weight 230

hgt 60 bmr<u>M</u> 1884 bmr<u>F</u> 1673 hgt 62 bmr<u>M</u> 1909 bmr<u>F</u> 1682
hgt 64 bmr<u>M</u> 1935 bmr<u>F</u> 1691 hgt 66 bmr<u>M</u> 1960 bmr<u>F</u> 1700
hgt 68 bmr<u>M</u> 1986 bmr<u>F</u> 1710 hgt 70 bmr<u>M</u> 2011 bmr<u>F</u> 1719
hgt 72 bmr<u>M</u> 2036 bmr<u>F</u> 1728 hgt 74 bmr<u>M</u> 2062 bmr<u>F</u> 1737
hgt 76 bmr<u>M</u> 2087 bmr<u>F</u> 1746 hgt 78 bmr<u>M</u> 2113 bmr<u>F</u> 1755

weight 240

hgt 60 bmr<u>M</u> 1946 bmr<u>F</u> 1717 hgt 62 bmr<u>M</u> 1972 bmr<u>F</u> 1726
hgt 64 bmr<u>M</u> 1997 bmr<u>F</u> 1735 hgt 66 bmr<u>M</u> 2022 bmr<u>F</u> 1744
hgt 68 bmr<u>M</u> 2048 bmr<u>F</u> 1753 hgt 70 bmr<u>M</u> 2073 bmr<u>F</u> 1762
hgt 72 bmr<u>M</u> 2099 bmr<u>F</u> 1771 hgt 74 bmr<u>M</u> 2124 bmr<u>F</u> 1781
hgt 76 bmr<u>M</u> 2149 bmr<u>F</u> 1790 hgt 78 bmr<u>M</u> 2175 bmr<u>F</u> 1799

weight 250

hgt 60 bmr<u>M</u> 2008 bmr<u>F</u> 1760 hgt 62 bmr<u>M</u> 2034 bmr<u>F</u> 1769
hgt 64 bmr<u>M</u> 2059 bmr<u>F</u> 1778 hgt 66 bmr<u>M</u> 2085 bmr<u>F</u> 1788
hgt 68 bmr<u>M</u> 2110 bmr<u>F</u> 1797 hgt 70 bmr<u>M</u> 2135 bmr<u>F</u> 1806
hgt 72 bmr<u>M</u> 2161 bmr<u>F</u> 1815 hgt 74 bmr<u>M</u> 2186 bmr<u>F</u> 1824
hgt 76 bmr<u>M</u> 2212 bmr<u>F</u> 1833 hgt 78 bmr<u>M</u> 2237 bmr<u>F</u> 1842

weight 260

hgt 60 bmr<u>M</u> 2071 bmr<u>F</u> 1804   hgt 62 bmr<u>M</u> 2096 bmr<u>F</u> 1813
hgt 64 bmr<u>M</u> 2121 bmr<u>F</u> 1822   hgt 66 bmr<u>M</u> 2147 bmr<u>F</u> 1831
hgt 68 bmr<u>M</u> 2172 bmr<u>F</u> 1840   hgt 70 bmr<u>M</u> 2198 bmr<u>F</u> 1850
hgt 72 bmr<u>M</u> 2223 bmr<u>F</u> 1859   hgt 74 bmr<u>M</u> 2248 bmr<u>F</u> 1868
hgt 76 bmr<u>M</u> 2274 bmr<u>F</u> 1877   hgt 78 bmr<u>M</u> 2299 bmr<u>F</u> 1886

weight 270

hgt 60 bmr<u>M</u> 2133 bmr<u>F</u> 1847   hgt 62 bmr<u>M</u> 2158 bmr<u>F</u> 1857
hgt 64 bmr<u>M</u> 2184 bmr<u>F</u> 1866   hgt 66 bmr<u>M</u> 2209 bmr<u>F</u> 1875
hgt 68 bmr<u>M</u> 2234 bmr<u>F</u> 1884   hgt 70 bmr<u>M</u> 2260 bmr<u>F</u> 1893
hgt 72 bmr<u>M</u> 2285 bmr<u>F</u> 1902   hgt 74 bmr<u>M</u> 2311 bmr<u>F</u> 1911
hgt 76 bmr<u>M</u> 2336 bmr<u>F</u> 1921   hgt 78 bmr<u>M</u> 2361 bmr<u>F</u> 1930

weight 280

hgt 60 bmr<u>M</u> 2195 bmr<u>F</u> 1891   hgt 62 bmr<u>M</u> 2220 bmr<u>F</u> 1900
hgt 64 bmr<u>M</u> 2246 bmr<u>F</u> 1909   hgt 66 bmr<u>M</u> 2271 bmr<u>F</u> 1918
hgt 68 bmr<u>M</u> 2297 bmr<u>F</u> 1928   hgt 70 bmr<u>M</u> 2322 bmr<u>F</u> 1937
hgt 72 bmr<u>M</u> 2347 bmr<u>F</u> 1946   hgt 74 bmr<u>M</u> 2373 bmr<u>F</u> 1955
hgt 76 bmr<u>M</u> 2398 bmr<u>F</u> 1964   hgt 78 bmr<u>M</u> 2424 bmr<u>F</u> 1973

weight 290

hgt 60 bmr<u>M</u> 2257 bmr<u>F</u> 1935   hgt 62 bmr<u>M</u> 2283 bmr<u>F</u> 1944
hgt 64 bmr<u>M</u> 2308 bmr<u>F</u> 1953   hgt 66 bmr<u>M</u> 2333 bmr<u>F</u> 1962
hgt 68 bmr<u>M</u> 2359 bmr<u>F</u> 1971   hgt 70 bmr<u>M</u> 2384 bmr<u>F</u> 1980
hgt 72 bmr<u>M</u> 2410 bmr<u>F</u> 1989   hgt 74 bmr<u>M</u> 2435 bmr<u>F</u> 1999
hgt 76 bmr<u>M</u> 2460 bmr<u>F</u> 2008   hgt 78 bmr<u>M</u> 2486 bmr<u>F</u> 2017

weight 300

hgt 60 bmr<u>M</u> 2319 bmr<u>F</u> 1978   hgt 62 bmr<u>M</u> 2345 bmr<u>F</u> 1987
hgt 64 bmr<u>M</u> 2370 bmr<u>F</u> 1996   hgt 66 bmr<u>M</u> 2396 bmr<u>F</u> 2006
hgt 68 bmr<u>M</u> 2421 bmr<u>F</u> 2015   hgt 70 bmr<u>M</u> 2446 bmr<u>F</u> 2024
hgt 72 bmr<u>M</u> 2472 bmr<u>F</u> 2033   hgt 74 bmr<u>M</u> 2497 bmr<u>F</u> 2042
hgt 76 bmr<u>M</u> 2523 bmr<u>F</u> 2051   hgt 78 bmr<u>M</u> 2548 bmr<u>F</u> 2060

Age 60

weight 110

hgt 60 bmr<u>M</u> 1104 bmr<u>F</u> 1126   hgt 62 bmr<u>M</u> 1129 bmr<u>F</u> 1135
hgt 64 bmr<u>M</u> 1154 bmr<u>F</u> 1145   hgt 66 bmr<u>M</u> 1180 bmr<u>F</u> 1154
hgt 68 bmr<u>M</u> 1205 bmr<u>F</u> 1163   hgt 70 bmr<u>M</u> 1231 bmr<u>F</u> 1172
hgt 72 bmr<u>M</u> 1256 bmr<u>F</u> 1181   hgt 74 bmr<u>M</u> 1281 bmr<u>F</u> 1190
hgt 76 bmr<u>M</u> 1307 bmr<u>F</u> 1199   hgt 78 bmr<u>M</u> 1332 bmr<u>F</u> 1209

<u>weight</u> 120

hgt 60 bmr<u>M</u> 1166 bmr<u>F</u> 1170   hgt 62 bmr<u>M</u> 1191 bmr<u>F</u> 1179
hgt 64 bmr<u>M</u> 1217 bmr<u>F</u> 1188   hgt 66 bmr<u>M</u> 1242 bmr<u>F</u> 1197
hgt 68 bmr<u>M</u> 1267 bmr<u>F</u> 1206   hgt 70 bmr<u>M</u> 1293 bmr<u>F</u> 1216
hgt 72 bmr<u>M</u> 1318 bmr<u>F</u> 1225   hgt 74 bmr<u>M</u> 1344 bmr<u>F</u> 1234
hgt 76 bmr<u>M</u> 1369 bmr<u>F</u> 1243   hgt 78 bmr<u>M</u> 1394 bmr<u>F</u> 1252

<u>weight</u> 130

hgt 60 bmr<u>M</u> 1228 bmr<u>F</u> 1214   hgt 62 bmr<u>M</u> 1253 bmr<u>F</u> 1223
hgt 64 bmr<u>M</u> 1279 bmr<u>F</u> 1232   hgt 66 bmr<u>M</u> 1304 bmr<u>F</u> 1241
hgt 68 bmr<u>M</u> 1330 bmr<u>F</u> 1250   hgt 70 bmr<u>M</u> 1355 bmr<u>F</u> 1259
hgt 72 bmr<u>M</u> 1380 bmr<u>F</u> 1268   hgt 74 bmr<u>M</u> 1406 bmr<u>F</u> 1277
hgt 76 bmr<u>M</u> 1431 bmr<u>F</u> 1287   hgt 78 bmr<u>M</u> 1457 bmr<u>F</u> 1296

<u>weight</u> 140

hgt 60 bmr<u>M</u> 1290 bmr<u>F</u> 1257   hgt 62 bmr<u>M</u> 1316 bmr<u>F</u> 1266
hgt 64 bmr<u>M</u> 1341 bmr<u>F</u> 1275   hgt 66 bmr<u>M</u> 1366 bmr<u>F</u> 1285
hgt 68 bmr<u>M</u> 1392 bmr<u>F</u> 1294   hgt 70 bmr<u>M</u> 1417 bmr<u>F</u> 1303
hgt 72 bmr<u>M</u> 1443 bmr<u>F</u> 1312   hgt 74 bmr<u>M</u> 1468 bmr<u>F</u> 1321
hgt 76 bmr<u>M</u> 1493 bmr<u>F</u> 1330   hgt 78 bmr<u>M</u> 1519 bmr<u>F</u> 1339

<u>weight</u> 150

hgt 60 bmr<u>M</u> 1352 bmr<u>F</u> 1301   hgt 62 bmr<u>M</u> 1378 bmr<u>F</u> 1310
hgt 64 bmr<u>M</u> 1403 bmr<u>F</u> 1319   hgt 66 bmr<u>M</u> 1429 bmr<u>F</u> 1328
hgt 68 bmr<u>M</u> 1454 bmr<u>F</u> 1337   hgt 70 bmr<u>M</u> 1479 bmr<u>F</u> 1346
hgt 72 bmr<u>M</u> 1505 bmr<u>F</u> 1356   hgt 74 bmr<u>M</u> 1530 bmr<u>F</u> 1365
hgt 76 bmr<u>M</u> 1556 bmr<u>F</u> 1374   hgt 78 bmr<u>M</u> 1581 bmr<u>F</u> 1383

<u>weight</u> 160

hgt 60 bmr<u>M</u> 1415 bmr<u>F</u> 1344   hgt 62 bmr<u>M</u> 1440 bmr<u>F</u> 1353
hgt 64 bmr<u>M</u> 1465 bmr<u>F</u> 1363   hgt 66 bmr<u>M</u> 1491 bmr<u>F</u> 1372
hgt 68 bmr<u>M</u> 1516 bmr<u>F</u> 1381   hgt 70 bmr<u>M</u> 1542 bmr<u>F</u> 1390
hgt 72 bmr<u>M</u> 1567 bmr<u>F</u> 1399   hgt 74 bmr<u>M</u> 1592 bmr<u>F</u> 1408
hgt 76 bmr<u>M</u> 1618 bmr<u>F</u> 1417   hgt 78 bmr<u>M</u> 1643 bmr<u>F</u> 1427

<u>weight</u> 170

hgt 60 bmr<u>M</u> 1477 bmr<u>F</u> 1388   hgt 62 bmr<u>M</u> 1502 bmr<u>F</u> 1397
hgt 64 bmr<u>M</u> 1528 bmr<u>F</u> 1406   hgt 66 bmr<u>M</u> 1553 bmr<u>F</u> 1415
hgt 68 bmr<u>M</u> 1578 bmr<u>F</u> 1424   hgt 70 bmr<u>M</u> 1604 bmr<u>F</u> 1434
hgt 72 bmr<u>M</u> 1629 bmr<u>F</u> 1443   hgt 74 bmr<u>M</u> 1655 bmr<u>F</u> 1452
hgt 76 bmr<u>M</u> 1680 bmr<u>F</u> 1461   hgt 78 bmr<u>M</u> 1705 bmr<u>F</u> 1470

weight 180

hgt 60 bmr<u>M</u> 1539 bmr<u>F</u> 1432   hgt 62 bmr<u>M</u> 1564 bmr<u>F</u> 1441
hgt 64 bmr<u>M</u> 1590 bmr<u>F</u> 1450   hgt 66 bmr<u>M</u> 1615 bmr<u>F</u> 1459
hgt 68 bmr<u>M</u> 1641 bmr<u>F</u> 1468   hgt 70 bmr<u>M</u> 1666 bmr<u>F</u> 1477
hgt 72 bmr<u>M</u> 1691 bmr<u>F</u> 1486   hgt 74 bmr<u>M</u> 1717 bmr<u>F</u> 1495
hgt 76 bmr<u>M</u> 1742 bmr<u>F</u> 1505   hgt 78 bmr<u>M</u> 1768 bmr<u>F</u> 1514

weight 190

hgt 60 bmr<u>M</u> 1601 bmr<u>F</u> 1475   hgt 62 bmr<u>M</u> 1627 bmr<u>F</u> 1484
hgt 64 bmr<u>M</u> 1652 bmr<u>F</u> 1493   hgt 66 bmr<u>M</u> 1677 bmr<u>F</u> 1503
hgt 68 bmr<u>M</u> 1703 bmr<u>F</u> 1512   hgt 70 bmr<u>M</u> 1728 bmr<u>F</u> 1521
hgt 72 bmr<u>M</u> 1754 bmr<u>F</u> 1530   hgt 74 bmr<u>M</u> 1779 bmr<u>F</u> 1539
hgt 76 bmr<u>M</u> 1804 bmr<u>F</u> 1548   hgt 78 bmr<u>M</u> 1830 bmr<u>F</u> 1557

weight 200

hgt 60 bmr<u>M</u> 1663 bmr<u>F</u> 1519   hgt 62 bmr<u>M</u> 1689 bmr<u>F</u> 1528
hgt 64 bmr<u>M</u> 1714 bmr<u>F</u> 1537   hgt 66 bmr<u>M</u> 1740 bmr<u>F</u> 1546
hgt 68 bmr<u>M</u> 1765 bmr<u>F</u> 1555   hgt 70 bmr<u>M</u> 1790 bmr<u>F</u> 1564
hgt 72 bmr<u>M</u> 1816 bmr<u>F</u> 1574   hgt 74 bmr<u>M</u> 1841 bmr<u>F</u> 1583
hgt 76 bmr<u>M</u> 1867 bmr<u>F</u> 1592   hgt 78 bmr<u>M</u> 1892 bmr<u>F</u> 1601

weight 210

hgt 60 bmr<u>M</u> 1726 bmr<u>F</u> 1562   hgt 62 bmr<u>M</u> 1751 bmr<u>F</u> 1571
hgt 64 bmr<u>M</u> 1776 bmr<u>F</u> 1581   hgt 66 bmr<u>M</u> 1802 bmr<u>F</u> 1590
hgt 68 bmr<u>M</u> 1827 bmr<u>F</u> 1599   hgt 70 bmr<u>M</u> 1853 bmr<u>F</u> 1608
hgt 72 bmr<u>M</u> 1878 bmr<u>F</u> 1617   hgt 74 bmr<u>M</u> 1903 bmr<u>F</u> 1626
hgt 76 bmr<u>M</u> 1929 bmr<u>F</u> 1635   hgt 78 bmr<u>M</u> 1954 bmr<u>F</u> 1645

weight 220

hgt 60 bmr<u>M</u> 1788 bmr<u>F</u> 1606   hgt 62 bmr<u>M</u> 1813 bmr<u>F</u> 1615
hgt 64 bmr<u>M</u> 1839 bmr<u>F</u> 1624   hgt 66 bmr<u>M</u> 1864 bmr<u>F</u> 1633
hgt 68 bmr<u>M</u> 1889 bmr<u>F</u> 1642   hgt 70 hmr<u>M</u> 1915 bmr<u>F</u> 1652
hgt 72 bmr<u>M</u> 1940 bmr<u>F</u> 1661   hgt 74 bmr<u>M</u> 1966 bmr<u>F</u> 1670
hgt 76 bmr<u>M</u> 1991 bmr<u>F</u> 1679   hgt 78 bmr<u>M</u> 2016 bmr<u>F</u> 1688

weight 230

hgt 60 bmr<u>M</u> 1850 bmr<u>F</u> 1650   hgt 62 bmr<u>M</u> 1875 bmr<u>F</u> 1659
hgt 64 bmr<u>M</u> 1901 bmr<u>F</u> 1668   hgt 66 bmr<u>M</u> 1926 bmr<u>F</u> 1677
hgt 68 bmr<u>M</u> 1952 bmr<u>F</u> 1686   hgt 70 bmr<u>M</u> 1977 bmr<u>F</u> 1695
hgt 72 bmr<u>M</u> 2002 bmr<u>F</u> 1704   hgt 74 bmr<u>M</u> 2028 bmr<u>F</u> 1713
hgt 76 bmr<u>M</u> 2053 bmr<u>F</u> 1723   hgt 78 bmr<u>M</u> 2079 bmr<u>F</u> 1732

weight 240

hgt 60 bmr<u>M</u> 1912 bmr<u>F</u> 1693   hgt 62 bmr<u>M</u> 1938 bmr<u>F</u> 1702
hgt 64 bmr<u>M</u> 1963 bmr<u>F</u> 1711   hgt 66 bmr<u>M</u> 1988 bmr<u>F</u> 1721
hgt 68 bmr<u>M</u> 2014 bmr<u>F</u> 1730   hgt 70 bmr<u>M</u> 2039 bmr<u>F</u> 1739
hgt 72 bmr<u>M</u> 2065 bmr<u>F</u> 1748   hgt 74 bmr<u>M</u> 2090 bmr<u>F</u> 1757
hgt 76 bmr<u>M</u> 2115 bmr<u>F</u> 1766   hgt 78 bmr<u>M</u> 2141 bmr<u>F</u> 1775

weight 250

hgt 60 bmr<u>M</u> 1974 bmr<u>F</u> 1737   hgt 62 bmr<u>M</u> 2000 bmr<u>F</u> 1746
hgt 64 bmr<u>M</u> 2025 bmr<u>F</u> 1755   hgt 66 bmr<u>M</u> 2051 bmr<u>F</u> 1764
hgt 68 bmr<u>M</u> 2076 bmr<u>F</u> 1773   hgt 70 bmr<u>M</u> 2101 bmr<u>F</u> 1782
hgt 72 bmr<u>M</u> 2127 bmr<u>F</u> 1792   hgt 74 bmr<u>M</u> 2152 bmr<u>F</u> 1801
hgt 76 bmr<u>M</u> 2178 bmr<u>F</u> 1810   hgt 78 bmr<u>M</u> 2203 bmr<u>F</u> 1819

weight 260

hgt 60 bmr<u>M</u> 2037 bmr<u>F</u> 1780   hgt 62 bmr<u>M</u> 2062 bmr<u>F</u> 1789
hgt 64 bmr<u>M</u> 2087 bmr<u>F</u> 1799   hgt 66 bmr<u>M</u> 2113 bmr<u>F</u> 1808
hgt 68 bmr<u>M</u> 2138 bmr<u>F</u> 1817   hgt 70 bmr<u>M</u> 2164 bmr<u>F</u> 1826
hgt 72 bmr<u>M</u> 2189 bmr<u>F</u> 1835   hgt 74 bmr<u>M</u> 2214 bmr<u>F</u> 1844
hgt 76 bmr<u>M</u> 2240 bmr<u>F</u> 1853   hgt 78 bmr<u>M</u> 2265 bmr<u>F</u> 1863

weight 270

hgt 60 bmr<u>M</u> 2099 bmr<u>F</u> 1824   hgt 62 bmr<u>M</u> 2124 bmr<u>F</u> 1833
hgt 64 bmr<u>M</u> 2150 bmr<u>F</u> 1842   hgt 66 bmr<u>M</u> 2175 bmr<u>F</u> 1851
hgt 68 bmr<u>M</u> 2200 bmr<u>F</u> 1860   hgt 70 bmr<u>M</u> 2226 bmr<u>F</u> 1870
hgt 72 bmr<u>M</u> 2251 bmr<u>F</u> 1879   hgt 74 bmr<u>M</u> 2277 bmr<u>F</u> 1888
hgt 76 bmr<u>M</u> 2302 bmr<u>F</u> 1897   hgt 78 bmr<u>M</u> 2327 bmr<u>F</u> 1906

weight 280

hgt 60 bmr<u>M</u> 2161 bmr<u>F</u> 1868   hgt 62 bmr<u>M</u> 2186 bmr<u>F</u> 1877
hgt 64 bmr<u>M</u> 2212 bmr<u>F</u> 1886   hgt 66 bmr<u>M</u> 2237 bmr<u>F</u> 1895
hgt 68 bmr<u>M</u> 2263 bmr<u>F</u> 1904   hgt 70 bmr<u>M</u> 2288 bmr<u>F</u> 1913
hgt 72 bmr<u>M</u> 2313 bmr<u>F</u> 1922   hgt 74 bmr<u>M</u> 2339 bmr<u>F</u> 1931
hgt 76 bmr<u>M</u> 2364 bmr<u>F</u> 1941   hgt 78 bmr<u>M</u> 2390 bmr<u>F</u> 1950

weight 290

hgt 60 bmr<u>M</u> 2223 bmr<u>F</u> 1911   hgt 62 bmr<u>M</u> 2249 bmr<u>F</u> 1920
hgt 64 bmr<u>M</u> 2274 bmr<u>F</u> 1929   hgt 66 bmr<u>M</u> 2299 bmr<u>F</u> 1939
hgt 68 bmr<u>M</u> 2325 bmr<u>F</u> 1948   hgt 70 bmr<u>M</u> 2350 bmr<u>F</u> 1957
hgt 72 bmr<u>M</u> 2376 bmr<u>F</u> 1966   hgt 74 bmr<u>M</u> 2401 bmr<u>F</u> 1975
hgt 76 bmr<u>M</u> 2426 bmr<u>F</u> 1984   hgt 78 bmr<u>M</u> 2452 bmr<u>F</u> 1993

weight 300

hgt 60	bmrM 2285	bmrF 1955	hgt 62	bmrM 2311	bmrF 1964
hgt 64	bmrM 2336	bmrF 1973	hgt 66	bmrM 2362	bmrF 1982
hgt 68	bmrM 2387	bmrF 1991	hgt 70	bmrM 2412	bmrF 2000
hgt 72	bmrM 2438	bmrF 2010	hgt 74	bmrM 2463	bmrF 2019
hgt 76	bmrM 2489	bmrF 2028	hgt 78	bmrM 2514	bmrF 2037

Age 65

weight 110

hgt 60	bmrM 1070	bmrF 1103	hgt 62	bmrM 1095	bmrF 1112
hgt 64	bmrM 1120	bmrF 1121	hgt 66	bmrM 1146	bmrF 1130
hgt 68	bmrM 1171	bmrF 1139	hgt 70	bmrM 1197	bmrF 1149
hgt 72	bmrM 1222	bmrF 1158	hgt 74	bmrM 1247	bmrF 1167
hgt 76	bmrM 1273	bmrF 1176	hgt 78	bmrM 1298	bmrF 1185

weight 120

hgt 60	bmrM 1132	bmrF 1146	hgt 62	bmrM 1157	bmrF 1156
hgt 64	bmrM 1183	bmrF 1165	hgt 66	bmrM 1208	bmrF 1174
hgt 68	bmrM 1233	bmrF 1183	hgt 70	bmrM 1259	bmrF 1192
hgt 72	bmrM 1284	bmrF 1201	hgt 74	bmrM 1310	bmrF 1210
hgt 76	bmrM 1335	bmrF 1220	hgt 78	bmrM 1360	bmrF 1229

weight 130

hgt 60	bmrM 1194	bmrF 1190	hgt 62	bmrM 1219	bmrF 1199
hgt 64	bmrM 1245	bmrF 1208	hgt 66	bmrM 1270	bmrF 1217
hgt 68	bmrM 1296	bmrF 1227	hgt 70	bmrM 1321	bmrF 1236
hgt 72	bmrM 1346	bmrF 1245	hgt 74	bmrM 1372	bmrF 1254
hgt 76	bmrM 1397	bmrF 1263	hgt 78	bmrM 1423	bmrF 1272

weight 140

hgt 60	bmrM 1256	bmrF 1234	hgt 62	bmrM 1282	bmrF 1243
hgt 64	bmrM 1307	bmrF 1252	hgt 66	bmrM 1332	bmrF 1261
hgt 68	bmrM 1358	bmrF 1270	hgt 70	bmrM 1383	bmrF 1279
hgt 72	bmrM 1409	bmrF 1288	hgt 74	bmrM 1434	bmrF 1298
hgt 76	bmrM 1459	bmrF 1307	hgt 78	bmrM 1485	bmrF 1316

weight 150

hgt 60	bmrM 1318	bmrF 1277	hgt 62	bmrM 1344	bmrF 1286
hgt 64	bmrM 1369	bmrF 1295	hgt 66	bmrM 1395	bmrF 1305
hgt 68	bmrM 1420	bmrF 1314	hgt 70	bmrM 1445	bmrF 1323
hgt 72	bmrM 1471	bmrF 1332	hgt 74	bmrM 1496	bmrF 1341
hgt 76	bmrM 1522	bmrF 1350	hgt 78	bmrM 1547	bmrF 1359

weight 160

hgt 60 bmr<u>M</u> 1381 bmr<u>F</u> 1321   hgt 62 bmr<u>M</u> 1406 bmr<u>F</u> 1330
hgt 64 bmr<u>M</u> 1431 bmr<u>F</u> 1339   hgt 66 bmr<u>M</u> 1457 bmr<u>F</u> 1348
hgt 68 bmr<u>M</u> 1482 bmr<u>F</u> 1357   hgt 70 bmr<u>M</u> 1508 bmr<u>F</u> 1367
hgt 72 bmr<u>M</u> 1533 bmr<u>F</u> 1376   hgt 74 bmr<u>M</u> 1558 bmr<u>F</u> 1385
hgt 76 bmr<u>M</u> 1584 bmr<u>F</u> 1394   hgt 78 bmr<u>M</u> 1609 bmr<u>F</u> 1403

weight 170

hgt 60 bmr<u>M</u> 1443 bmr<u>F</u> 1364   hgt 62 bmr<u>M</u> 1468 bmr<u>F</u> 1374
hgt 64 bmr<u>M</u> 1494 bmr<u>F</u> 1383   hgt 66 bmr<u>M</u> 1519 bmr<u>F</u> 1392
hgt 68 bmr<u>M</u> 1544 bmr<u>F</u> 1401   hgt 70 bmr<u>M</u> 1570 bmr<u>F</u> 1410
hgt 72 bmr<u>M</u> 1595 bmr<u>F</u> 1419   hgt 74 bmr<u>M</u> 1621 bmr<u>F</u> 1428
hgt 76 bmr<u>M</u> 1646 bmr<u>F</u> 1438   hgt 78 bmr<u>M</u> 1671 bmr<u>F</u> 1447

weight 180

hgt 60 bmr<u>M</u> 1505 bmr<u>F</u> 1408   hgt 62 bmr<u>M</u> 1530 bmr<u>F</u> 1417
hgt 64 bmr<u>M</u> 1556 bmr<u>F</u> 1426   hgt 66 bmr<u>M</u> 1581 bmr<u>F</u> 1435
hgt 68 bmr<u>M</u> 1607 bmr<u>F</u> 1445   hgt 70 bmr<u>M</u> 1632 bmr<u>F</u> 1454
hgt 72 bmr<u>M</u> 1657 bmr<u>F</u> 1463   hgt 74 bmr<u>M</u> 1683 bmr<u>F</u> 1472
hgt 76 bmr<u>M</u> 1708 bmr<u>F</u> 1481   hgt 78 bmr<u>M</u> 1734 bmr<u>F</u> 1490

weight 190

hgt 60 bmr<u>M</u> 1567 bmr<u>F</u> 1452   hgt 62 bmr<u>M</u> 1593 bmr<u>F</u> 1461
hgt 64 bmr<u>M</u> 1618 bmr<u>F</u> 1470   hgt 66 bmr<u>M</u> 1643 bmr<u>F</u> 1479
hgt 68 bmr<u>M</u> 1669 bmr<u>F</u> 1488   hgt 70 bmr<u>M</u> 1694 bmr<u>F</u> 1497
hgt 72 bmr<u>M</u> 1720 bmr<u>F</u> 1506   hgt 74 bmr<u>M</u> 1745 bmr<u>F</u> 1516
hgt 76 bmr<u>M</u> 1770 bmr<u>F</u> 1525   hgt 78 bmr<u>M</u> 1796 bmr<u>F</u> 1534

weight 200

hgt 60 bmr<u>M</u> 1629 bmr<u>F</u> 1495   hgt 62 bmr<u>M</u> 1655 bmr<u>F</u> 1504
hgt 64 bmr<u>M</u> 1680 bmr<u>F</u> 1513   hgt 66 bmr<u>M</u> 1706 bmr<u>F</u> 1523
hgt 68 bmr<u>M</u> 1731 bmr<u>F</u> 1532   hgt 70 bmr<u>M</u> 1756 bmr<u>F</u> 1541
hgt 72 bmr<u>M</u> 1782 bmr<u>F</u> 1550   hgt 74 bmr<u>M</u> 1807 bmr<u>F</u> 1559
hgt 76 bmr<u>M</u> 1833 bmr<u>F</u> 1568   hgt 78 bmr<u>M</u> 1858 bmr<u>F</u> 1577

weight 210

hgt 60 bmr<u>M</u> 1692 bmr<u>F</u> 1539   hgt 62 bmr<u>M</u> 1717 bmr<u>F</u> 1548
hgt 64 bmr<u>M</u> 1742 bmr<u>F</u> 1557   hgt 66 bmr<u>M</u> 1768 bmr<u>F</u> 1566
hgt 68 bmr<u>M</u> 1793 bmr<u>F</u> 1575   hgt 70 bmr<u>M</u> 1819 bmr<u>F</u> 1585
hgt 72 bmr<u>M</u> 1844 bmr<u>F</u> 1594   hgt 74 bmr<u>M</u> 1869 bmr<u>F</u> 1603
hgt 76 bmr<u>M</u> 1895 bmr<u>F</u> 1612   hgt 78 bmr<u>M</u> 1920 bmr<u>F</u> 1621

weight 220

hgt 60 bmr<u>M</u> 1754 bmr<u>F</u> 1582 hgt 62 bmr<u>M</u> 1779 bmr<u>F</u> 1592
hgt 64 bmr<u>M</u> 1805 bmr<u>F</u> 1601 hgt 66 bmr<u>M</u> 1830 bmr<u>F</u> 1610
hgt 68 bmr<u>M</u> 1855 bmr<u>F</u> 1619 hgt 70 bmr<u>M</u> 1881 bmr<u>F</u> 1628
hgt 72 bmr<u>M</u> 1906 bmr<u>F</u> 1637 hgt 74 bmr<u>M</u> 1932 bmr<u>F</u> 1646
hgt 76 bmr<u>M</u> 1957 bmr<u>F</u> 1656 hgt 78 bmr<u>M</u> 1982 bmr<u>F</u> 1665

weight 230

hgt 60 bmr<u>M</u> 1816 bmr<u>F</u> 1626 hgt 62 bmr<u>M</u> 1841 bmr<u>F</u> 1635
hgt 64 bmr<u>M</u> 1867 bmr<u>F</u> 1644 hgt 66 bmr<u>M</u> 1892 bmr<u>F</u> 1653
hgt 68 bmr<u>M</u> 1918 bmr<u>F</u> 1663 hgt 70 bmr<u>M</u> 1943 bmr<u>F</u> 1672
hgt 72 bmr<u>M</u> 1968 bmr<u>F</u> 1681 hgt 74 bmr<u>M</u> 1994 bmr<u>F</u> 1690
hgt 76 bmr<u>M</u> 2019 bmr<u>F</u> 1699 hgt 78 bmr<u>M</u> 2045 bmr<u>F</u> 1708

weight 240

hgt 60 bmr<u>M</u> 1878 bmr<u>F</u> 1670 hgt 62 bmr<u>M</u> 1904 bmr<u>F</u> 1679
hgt 64 bmr<u>M</u> 1929 bmr<u>F</u> 1688 hgt 66 bmr<u>M</u> 1954 bmr<u>F</u> 1697
hgt 68 bmr<u>M</u> 1980 bmr<u>F</u> 1706 hgt 70 bmr<u>M</u> 2005 bmr<u>F</u> 1715
hgt 72 bmr<u>M</u> 2031 bmr<u>F</u> 1724 hgt 74 bmr<u>M</u> 2056 bmr<u>F</u> 1734
hgt 76 bmr<u>M</u> 2081 bmr<u>F</u> 1743 hgt 78 bmr<u>M</u> 2107 bmr<u>F</u> 1752

weight 250

hgt 60 bmr<u>M</u> 1940 bmr<u>F</u> 1713 hgt 62 bmr<u>M</u> 1966 bmr<u>F</u> 1722
hgt 64 bmr<u>M</u> 1991 bmr<u>F</u> 1731 hgt 66 bmr<u>M</u> 2017 bmr<u>F</u> 1741
hgt 68 bmr<u>M</u> 2042 bmr<u>F</u> 1750 hgt 70 bmr<u>M</u> 2067 bmr<u>F</u> 1759
hgt 72 bmr<u>M</u> 2093 bmr<u>F</u> 1768 hgt 74 bmr<u>M</u> 2118 bmr<u>F</u> 1777
hgt 76 bmr<u>M</u> 2144 bmr<u>F</u> 1786 hgt 78 bmr<u>M</u> 2169 bmr<u>F</u> 1795

weight 260

hgt 60 bmr<u>M</u> 2003 bmr<u>F</u> 1757 hgt 62 bmr<u>M</u> 2028 bmr<u>F</u> 1766
hgt 64 bmr<u>M</u> 2053 bmr<u>F</u> 1775 hgt 66 bmr<u>M</u> 2079 bmr<u>F</u> 1784
hgt 68 bmr<u>M</u> 2104 bmr<u>F</u> 1793 hgt 70 bmr<u>M</u> 2130 bmr<u>F</u> 1803
hgt 72 bmr<u>M</u> 2155 bmr<u>F</u> 1812 hgt 74 bmr<u>M</u> 2180 bmr<u>F</u> 1821
hgt 76 bmr<u>M</u> 2206 bmr<u>F</u> 1830 hgt 78 bmr<u>M</u> 2231 bmr<u>F</u> 1839

weight 270

hgt 60 bmr<u>M</u> 2065 bmr<u>F</u> 1800 hgt 62 bmr<u>M</u> 2090 bmr<u>F</u> 1810
hgt 64 bmr<u>M</u> 2116 bmr<u>F</u> 1819 hgt 66 bmr<u>M</u> 2141 bmr<u>F</u> 1828
hgt 68 bmr<u>M</u> 2166 bmr<u>F</u> 1837 hgt 70 bmr<u>M</u> 2192 bmr<u>F</u> 1846
hgt 72 bmr<u>M</u> 2217 bmr<u>F</u> 1855 hgt 74 bmr<u>M</u> 2243 bmr<u>F</u> 1864
hgt 76 bmr<u>M</u> 2268 bmr<u>F</u> 1874 hgt 78 bmr<u>M</u> 2293 bmr<u>F</u> 1883

<u>weight</u> 280

hgt 60 bmr<u>M</u> 2127 bmr<u>F</u> 1844   hgt 62 bmr<u>M</u> 2152 bmr<u>F</u> 1853
hgt 64 bmr<u>M</u> 2178 bmr<u>F</u> 1862   hgt 66 bmr<u>M</u> 2203 bmr<u>F</u> 1871
hgt 68 bmr<u>M</u> 2229 bmr<u>F</u> 1881   hgt 70 bmr<u>M</u> 2254 bmr<u>F</u> 1890
hgt 72 bmr<u>M</u> 2279 bmr<u>F</u> 1899   hgt 74 bmr<u>M</u> 2305 bmr<u>F</u> 1908
hgt 76 bmr<u>M</u> 2330 bmr<u>F</u> 1917   hgt 78 bmr<u>M</u> 2356 bmr<u>F</u> 1926

<u>weight</u> 290

hgt 60 bmr<u>M</u> 2189 bmr<u>F</u> 1888   hgt 62 bmr<u>M</u> 2215 bmr<u>F</u> 1897
hgt 64 bmr<u>M</u> 2240 bmr<u>F</u> 1906   hgt 66 bmr<u>M</u> 2265 bmr<u>F</u> 1915
hgt 68 bmr<u>M</u> 2291 bmr<u>F</u> 1924   hgt 70 bmr<u>M</u> 2316 bmr<u>F</u> 1933
hgt 72 bmr<u>M</u> 2342 bmr<u>F</u> 1942   hgt 74 bmr<u>M</u> 2367 bmr<u>F</u> 1952
hgt 76 bmr<u>M</u> 2392 bmr<u>F</u> 1961   hgt 78 bmr<u>M</u> 2418 bmr<u>F</u> 1970

<u>weight</u> 300

hgt 60 bmr<u>M</u> 2251 bmr<u>F</u> 1931   hgt 62 bmr<u>M</u> 2277 bmr<u>F</u> 1940
hgt 64 bmr<u>M</u> 2302 bmr<u>F</u> 1949   hgt 66 bmr<u>M</u> 2328 bmr<u>F</u> 1959
hgt 68 bmr<u>M</u> 2353 bmr<u>F</u> 1968   hgt 70 bmr<u>M</u> 2378 bmr<u>F</u> 1977
hgt 72 bmr<u>M</u> 2404 bmr<u>F</u> 1986   hgt 74 bmr<u>M</u> 2429 bmr<u>F</u> 1995
hgt 76 bmr<u>M</u> 2455 bmr<u>F</u> 2004   hgt 78 bmr<u>M</u> 2480 bmr<u>F</u> 2013

Age 70

<u>weight</u> 110

hgt 60 bmr<u>M</u> 1036 bmr<u>F</u> 1079   hgt 62 bmr<u>M</u> 1061 bmr<u>F</u> 1088
hgt 64 bmr<u>M</u> 1086 bmr<u>F</u> 1098   hgt 66 bmr<u>M</u> 1112 bmr<u>F</u> 1107
hgt 68 bmr<u>M</u> 1137 bmr<u>F</u> 1116   hgt 70 bmr<u>M</u> 1163 bmr<u>F</u> 1125
hgt 72 bmr<u>M</u> 1188 bmr<u>F</u> 1134   hgt 74 bmr<u>M</u> 1213 bmr<u>F</u> 1143
hgt 76 bmr<u>M</u> 1239 bmr<u>F</u> 1152   hgt 78 bmr<u>M</u> 1264 bmr<u>F</u> 1162

<u>weight</u> 120

hgt 60 bmr<u>M</u> 1098 bmr<u>F</u> 1123   hgt 62 bmr<u>M</u> 1123 bmr<u>F</u> 1132
hgt 64 bmr<u>M</u> 1149 bmr<u>F</u> 1141   hgt 66 bmr<u>M</u> 1174 bmr<u>F</u> 1150
hgt 68 bmr<u>M</u> 1199 bmr<u>F</u> 1159   hgt 70 bmr<u>M</u> 1225 bmr<u>F</u> 1169
hgt 72 bmr<u>M</u> 1250 bmr<u>F</u> 1178   hgt 74 bmr<u>M</u> 1276 bmr<u>F</u> 1187
hgt 76 bmr<u>M</u> 1301 bmr<u>F</u> 1196   hgt 78 bmr<u>M</u> 1326 bmr<u>F</u> 1205

<u>weight</u> 130

hgt 60 bmr<u>M</u> 1160 bmr<u>F</u> 1167   hgt 62 bmr<u>M</u> 1185 bmr<u>F</u> 1176
hgt 64 bmr<u>M</u> 1211 bmr<u>F</u> 1185   hgt 66 bmr<u>M</u> 1236 bmr<u>F</u> 1194
hgt 68 bmr<u>M</u> 1262 bmr<u>F</u> 1203   hgt 70 bmr<u>M</u> 1287 bmr<u>F</u> 1212
hgt 72 bmr<u>M</u> 1312 bmr<u>F</u> 1221   hgt 74 bmr<u>M</u> 1338 bmr<u>F</u> 1230
hgt 76 bmr<u>M</u> 1363 bmr<u>F</u> 1240   hgt 78 bmr<u>M</u> 1389 bmr<u>F</u> 1249

<u>weight</u> 140

hgt 60 bmr<u>M</u> 1222 bmr<u>F</u> 1210   hgt 62 bmr<u>M</u> 1248 bmr<u>F</u> 1219
hgt 64 bmr<u>M</u> 1273 bmr<u>F</u> 1228   hgt 66 bmr<u>M</u> 1298 bmr<u>F</u> 1238
hgt 68 bmr<u>M</u> 1324 bmr<u>F</u> 1247   hgt 70 bmr<u>M</u> 1349 bmr<u>F</u> 1256
hgt 72 bmr<u>M</u> 1375 bmr<u>F</u> 1265   hgt 74 bmr<u>M</u> 1400 bmr<u>F</u> 1274
hgt 76 bmr<u>M</u> 1425 bmr<u>F</u> 1283   hgt 78 bmr<u>M</u> 1451 bmr<u>F</u> 1292

<u>weight</u> 150

hgt 60 bmr<u>M</u> 1284 bmr<u>F</u> 1254   hgt 62 bmr<u>M</u> 1310 bmr<u>F</u> 1263
hgt 64 bmr<u>M</u> 1335 bmr<u>F</u> 1272   hgt 66 bmr<u>M</u> 1361 bmr<u>F</u> 1281
hgt 68 bmr<u>M</u> 1386 bmr<u>F</u> 1290   hgt 70 bmr<u>M</u> 1411 bmr<u>F</u> 1299
hgt 72 bmr<u>M</u> 1437 bmr<u>F</u> 1309   hgt 74 bmr<u>M</u> 1462 bmr<u>F</u> 1318
hgt 76 bmr<u>M</u> 1488 bmr<u>F</u> 1327   hgt 78 bmr<u>M</u> 1513 bmr<u>F</u> 1336

<u>weight</u> 160

hgt 60 bmr<u>M</u> 1347 bmr<u>F</u> 1297   hgt 62 bmr<u>M</u> 1372 bmr<u>F</u> 1306
hgt 64 bmr<u>M</u> 1397 bmr<u>F</u> 1316   hgt 66 bmr<u>M</u> 1423 bmr<u>F</u> 1325
hgt 68 bmr<u>M</u> 1448 bmr<u>F</u> 1334   hgt 70 bmr<u>M</u> 1474 bmr<u>F</u> 1343
hgt 72 bmr<u>M</u> 1499 bmr<u>F</u> 1352   hgt 74 bmr<u>M</u> 1524 bmr<u>F</u> 1361
hgt 76 bmr<u>M</u> 1550 bmr<u>F</u> 1370   hgt 78 bmr<u>M</u> 1575 bmr<u>F</u> 1380

<u>weight</u> 170

hgt 60 bmr<u>M</u> 1409 bmr<u>F</u> 1341   hgt 62 bmr<u>M</u> 1434 bmr<u>F</u> 1350
hgt 64 bmr<u>M</u> 1460 bmr<u>F</u> 1359   hgt 66 bmr<u>M</u> 1485 bmr<u>F</u> 1368
hgt 68 bmr<u>M</u> 1510 bmr<u>F</u> 1377   hgt 70 bmr<u>M</u> 1536 bmr<u>F</u> 1387
hgt 72 bmr<u>M</u> 1561 bmr<u>F</u> 1396   hgt 74 bmr<u>M</u> 1587 bmr<u>F</u> 1405
hgt 76 bmr<u>M</u> 1612 bmr<u>F</u> 1414   hgt 78 bmr<u>M</u> 1637 bmr<u>F</u> 1423

<u>weight</u> 180

hgt 60 bmr<u>M</u> 1471 bmr<u>F</u> 1385   hgt 62 bmr<u>M</u> 1496 bmr<u>F</u> 1394
hgt 64 bmr<u>M</u> 1522 bmr<u>F</u> 1403   hgt 66 bmr<u>M</u> 1547 bmr<u>F</u> 1412
hgt 68 bmr<u>M</u> 1573 bmr<u>F</u> 1421   hgt 70 hmr<u>M</u> 1598 bmr<u>F</u> 1430
hgt 72 bmr<u>M</u> 1623 bmr<u>F</u> 1439   hgt 74 bmr<u>M</u> 1649 bmr<u>F</u> 1448
hgt 76 bmr<u>M</u> 1674 bmr<u>F</u> 1458   hgt 78 bmr<u>M</u> 1700 bmr<u>F</u> 1467

<u>weight</u> 190

hgt 60 bmr<u>M</u> 1533 bmr<u>F</u> 1428   hgt 62 bmr<u>M</u> 1559 bmr<u>F</u> 1437
hgt 64 bmr<u>M</u> 1584 bmr<u>F</u> 1446   hgt 66 bmr<u>M</u> 1609 bmr<u>F</u> 1456
hgt 68 bmr<u>M</u> 1635 bmr<u>F</u> 1465   hgt 70 bmr<u>M</u> 1660 bmr<u>F</u> 1474
hgt 72 bmr<u>M</u> 1686 bmr<u>F</u> 1483   hgt 74 bmr<u>M</u> 1711 bmr<u>F</u> 1492
hgt 76 bmr<u>M</u> 1736 bmr<u>F</u> 1501   hgt 78 bmr<u>M</u> 1762 bmr<u>F</u> 1510

weight 200

hgt 60 bmr<u>M</u> 1595 bmr<u>F</u> 1472   hgt 62 bmr<u>M</u> 1621 bmr<u>F</u> 1481
hgt 64 bmr<u>M</u> 1646 bmr<u>F</u> 1490   hgt 66 bmr<u>M</u> 1672 bmr<u>F</u> 1499
hgt 68 bmr<u>M</u> 1697 bmr<u>F</u> 1508   hgt 70 bmr<u>M</u> 1722 bmr<u>F</u> 1517
hgt 72 bmr<u>M</u> 1748 bmr<u>F</u> 1527   hgt 74 bmr<u>M</u> 1773 bmr<u>F</u> 1536
hgt 76 bmr<u>M</u> 1799 bmr<u>F</u> 1545   hgt 78 bmr<u>M</u> 1824 bmr<u>F</u> 1554

weight 210

hgt 60 bmr<u>M</u> 1658 bmr<u>F</u> 1515   hgt 62 bmr<u>M</u> 1683 bmr<u>F</u> 1524
hgt 64 bmr<u>M</u> 1708 bmr<u>F</u> 1534   hgt 66 bmr<u>M</u> 1734 bmr<u>F</u> 1543
hgt 68 bmr<u>M</u> 1759 bmr<u>F</u> 1552   hgt 70 bmr<u>M</u> 1785 bmr<u>F</u> 1561
hgt 72 bmr<u>M</u> 1810 bmr<u>F</u> 1570   hgt 74 bmr<u>M</u> 1835 bmr<u>F</u> 1579
hgt 76 bmr<u>M</u> 1861 bmr<u>F</u> 1588   hgt 78 bmr<u>M</u> 1886 bmr<u>F</u> 1598

weight 220

hgt 60 bmr<u>M</u> 1720 bmr<u>F</u> 1559   hgt 62 bmr<u>M</u> 1745 bmr<u>F</u> 1568
hgt 64 bmr<u>M</u> 1771 bmr<u>F</u> 1577   hgt 66 bmr<u>M</u> 1796 bmr<u>F</u> 1586
hgt 68 bmr<u>M</u> 1821 bmr<u>F</u> 1595   hgt 70 bmr<u>M</u> 1847 bmr<u>F</u> 1605
hgt 72 bmr<u>M</u> 1872 bmr<u>F</u> 1614   hgt 74 bmr<u>M</u> 1898 bmr<u>F</u> 1623
hgt 76 bmr<u>M</u> 1923 bmr<u>F</u> 1632   hgt 78 bmr<u>M</u> 1948 bmr<u>F</u> 1641

weight 230

hgt 60 bmr<u>M</u> 1782 bmr<u>F</u> 1603   hgt 62 bmr<u>M</u> 1807 bmr<u>F</u> 1612
hgt 64 bmr<u>M</u> 1833 bmr<u>F</u> 1621   hgt 66 bmr<u>M</u> 1858 bmr<u>F</u> 1630
hgt 68 bmr<u>M</u> 1884 bmr<u>F</u> 1639   hgt 70 bmr<u>M</u> 1909 bmr<u>F</u> 1648
hgt 72 bmr<u>M</u> 1934 bmr<u>F</u> 1657   hgt 74 bmr<u>M</u> 1960 bmr<u>F</u> 1666
hgt 76 bmr<u>M</u> 1985 bmr<u>F</u> 1676   hgt 78 bmr<u>M</u> 2011 bmr<u>F</u> 1685

weight 240

hgt 60 bmr<u>M</u> 1844 bmr<u>F</u> 1646   hgt 62 bmr<u>M</u> 1870 bmr<u>F</u> 1655
hgt 64 bmr<u>M</u> 1895 bmr<u>F</u> 1664   hgt 66 bmr<u>M</u> 1920 bmr<u>F</u> 1674
hgt 68 bmr<u>M</u> 1946 bmr<u>F</u> 1683   hgt 70 bmr<u>M</u> 1971 bmr<u>F</u> 1692
hgt 72 bmr<u>M</u> 1997 bmr<u>F</u> 1701   hgt 74 bmr<u>M</u> 2022 bmr<u>F</u> 1710
hgt 76 bmr<u>M</u> 2047 bmr<u>F</u> 1719   hgt 78 bmr<u>M</u> 2073 bmr<u>F</u> 1728

weight 250

hgt 60 bmr<u>M</u> 1906 bmr<u>F</u> 1690   hgt 62 bmr<u>M</u> 1932 bmr<u>F</u> 1699
hgt 64 bmr<u>M</u> 1957 bmr<u>F</u> 1708   hgt 66 bmr<u>M</u> 1983 bmr<u>F</u> 1717
hgt 68 bmr<u>M</u> 2008 bmr<u>F</u> 1726   hgt 70 bmr<u>M</u> 2033 bmr<u>F</u> 1735
hgt 72 bmr<u>M</u> 2059 bmr<u>F</u> 1745   hgt 74 bmr<u>M</u> 2084 bmr<u>F</u> 1754
hgt 76 bmr<u>M</u> 2110 bmr<u>F</u> 1763   hgt 78 bmr<u>M</u> 2135 bmr<u>F</u> 1772

weight 260

hgt 60 bmr<u>M</u> 1969 bmr<u>F</u> 1733   hgt 62 bmr<u>M</u> 1994 bmr<u>F</u> 1742
hgt 64 bmr<u>M</u> 2019 bmr<u>F</u> 1752   hgt 66 bmr<u>M</u> 2045 bmr<u>F</u> 1761
hgt 68 bmr<u>M</u> 2070 bmr<u>F</u> 1770   hgt 70 bmr<u>M</u> 2096 bmr<u>F</u> 1779
hgt 72 bmr<u>M</u> 2121 bmr<u>F</u> 1788   hgt 74 bmr<u>M</u> 2146 bmr<u>F</u> 1797
hgt 76 bmr<u>M</u> 2172 bmr<u>F</u> 1806   hgt 78 bmr<u>M</u> 2197 bmr<u>F</u> 1816

weight 270

hgt 60 bmr<u>M</u> 2031 bmr<u>F</u> 1777   hgt 62 bmr<u>M</u> 2056 bmr<u>F</u> 1786
hgt 64 bmr<u>M</u> 2082 bmr<u>F</u> 1795   hgt 66 bmr<u>M</u> 2107 bmr<u>F</u> 1804
hgt 68 bmr<u>M</u> 2132 bmr<u>F</u> 1813   hgt 70 bmr<u>M</u> 2158 bmr<u>F</u> 1823
hgt 72 bmr<u>M</u> 2183 bmr<u>F</u> 1832   hgt 74 bmr<u>M</u> 2209 bmr<u>F</u> 1841
hgt 76 bmr<u>M</u> 2234 bmr<u>F</u> 1850   hgt 78 bmr<u>M</u> 2259 bmr<u>F</u> 1859

weight 280

hgt 60 bmr<u>M</u> 2093 bmr<u>F</u> 1821   hgt 62 bmr<u>M</u> 2118 bmr<u>F</u> 1830
hgt 64 bmr<u>M</u> 2144 bmr<u>F</u> 1839   hgt 66 bmr<u>M</u> 2169 bmr<u>F</u> 1848
hgt 68 bmr<u>M</u> 2195 bmr<u>F</u> 1857   hgt 70 bmr<u>M</u> 2220 bmr<u>F</u> 1866
hgt 72 bmr<u>M</u> 2245 bmr<u>F</u> 1875   hgt 74 bmr<u>M</u> 2271 bmr<u>F</u> 1884
hgt 76 bmr<u>M</u> 2296 bmr<u>F</u> 1894   hgt 78 bmr<u>M</u> 2322 bmr<u>F</u> 1903

weight 290

hgt 60 bmr<u>M</u> 2155 bmr<u>F</u> 1864   hgt 62 bmr<u>M</u> 2181 bmr<u>F</u> 1873
hgt 64 bmr<u>M</u> 2206 bmr<u>F</u> 1882   hgt 66 bmr<u>M</u> 2231 bmr<u>F</u> 1892
hgt 68 bmr<u>M</u> 2257 bmr<u>F</u> 1901   hgt 70 bmr<u>M</u> 2282 bmr<u>F</u> 1910
hgt 72 bmr<u>M</u> 2308 bmr<u>F</u> 1919   hgt 74 bmr<u>M</u> 2333 bmr<u>F</u> 1928
hgt 76 bmr<u>M</u> 2358 bmr<u>F</u> 1937   hgt 78 bmr<u>M</u> 2384 bmr<u>F</u> 1946

weight 300

hgt 60 bmr<u>M</u> 2217 bmr<u>F</u> 1908   hgt 62 bmr<u>M</u> 2243 bmr<u>F</u> 1917
hgt 64 bmr<u>M</u> 2268 bmr<u>F</u> 1926   hgt 66 bmr<u>M</u> 2294 bmr<u>F</u> 1935
hgt 68 bmr<u>M</u> 2319 bmr<u>F</u> 1944   hgt 70 bmr<u>M</u> 2344 hmr<u>F</u> 1953
hgt 72 bmr<u>M</u> 2370 bmr<u>F</u> 1963   hgt 74 bmr<u>M</u> 2395 bmr<u>F</u> 1972
hgt 76 bmr<u>M</u> 2421 bmr<u>F</u> 1981   hgt 78 bmr<u>M</u> 2446 bmr<u>F</u> 1990

Age 75

weight 110

hgt 60 bmr<u>M</u> 1002 bmr<u>F</u> 1056   hgt 62 bmr<u>M</u> 1027 bmr<u>F</u> 1065
hgt 64 bmr<u>M</u> 1052 bmr<u>F</u> 1074   hgt 66 bmr<u>M</u> 1078 bmr<u>F</u> 1083
hgt 68 bmr<u>M</u> 1103 bmr<u>F</u> 1092   hgt 70 bmr<u>M</u> 1129 bmr<u>F</u> 1102
hgt 72 bmr<u>M</u> 1154 bmr<u>F</u> 1111   hgt 74 bmr<u>M</u> 1179 bmr<u>F</u> 1120
hgt 76 bmr<u>M</u> 1205 bmr<u>F</u> 1129   hgt 78 bmr<u>M</u> 1230 bmr<u>F</u> 1138

weight 120

hgt 60 bmr<u>M</u> 1064 bmr<u>F</u> 1099 hgt 62 bmr<u>M</u> 1089 bmr<u>F</u> 1109
hgt 64 bmr<u>M</u> 1115 bmr<u>F</u> 1118 hgt 66 bmr<u>M</u> 1140 bmr<u>F</u> 1127
hgt 68 bmr<u>M</u> 1165 bmr<u>F</u> 1136 hgt 70 bmr<u>M</u> 1191 bmr<u>F</u> 1145
hgt 72 bmr<u>M</u> 1216 bmr<u>F</u> 1154 hgt 74 bmr<u>M</u> 1242 bmr<u>F</u> 1163
hgt 76 bmr<u>M</u> 1267 bmr<u>F</u> 1173 hgt 78 bmr<u>M</u> 1292 bmr<u>F</u> 1182

weight 130

hgt 60 bmr<u>M</u> 1126 bmr<u>F</u> 1143 hgt 62 bmr<u>M</u> 1151 bmr<u>F</u> 1152
hgt 64 bmr<u>M</u> 1177 bmr<u>F</u> 1161 hgt 66 bmr<u>M</u> 1202 bmr<u>F</u> 1170
hgt 68 bmr<u>M</u> 1228 bmr<u>F</u> 1180 hgt 70 bmr<u>M</u> 1253 bmr<u>F</u> 1189
hgt 72 bmr<u>M</u> 1278 bmr<u>F</u> 1198 hgt 74 bmr<u>M</u> 1304 bmr<u>F</u> 1207
hgt 76 bmr<u>M</u> 1329 bmr<u>F</u> 1216 hgt 78 bmr<u>M</u> 1355 bmr<u>F</u> 1225

weight 140

hgt 60 bmr<u>M</u> 1188 bmr<u>F</u> 1187 hgt 62 bmr<u>M</u> 1214 bmr<u>F</u> 1196
hgt 64 bmr<u>M</u> 1239 bmr<u>F</u> 1205 hgt 66 bmr<u>M</u> 1264 bmr<u>F</u> 1214
hgt 68 bmr<u>M</u> 1290 bmr<u>F</u> 1223 hgt 70 bmr<u>M</u> 1315 bmr<u>F</u> 1232
hgt 72 bmr<u>M</u> 1341 bmr<u>F</u> 1241 hgt 74 bmr<u>M</u> 1366 bmr<u>F</u> 1251
hgt 76 bmr<u>M</u> 1391 bmr<u>F</u> 1260 hgt 78 bmr<u>M</u> 1417 bmr<u>F</u> 1269

weight 150

hgt 60 bmr<u>M</u> 1250 bmr<u>F</u> 1230 hgt 62 bmr<u>M</u> 1276 bmr<u>F</u> 1239
hgt 64 bmr<u>M</u> 1301 bmr<u>F</u> 1248 hgt 66 bmr<u>M</u> 1327 bmr<u>F</u> 1258
hgt 68 bmr<u>M</u> 1352 bmr<u>F</u> 1267 hgt 70 bmr<u>M</u> 1377 bmr<u>F</u> 1276
hgt 72 bmr<u>M</u> 1403 bmr<u>F</u> 1285 hgt 74 bmr<u>M</u> 1428 bmr<u>F</u> 1294
hgt 76 bmr<u>M</u> 1454 bmr<u>F</u> 1303 hgt 78 bmr<u>M</u> 1479 bmr<u>F</u> 1312

weight 160

hgt 60 bmr<u>M</u> 1313 bmr<u>F</u> 1274 hgt 62 bmr<u>M</u> 1338 bmr<u>F</u> 1283
hgt 64 bmr<u>M</u> 1363 bmr<u>F</u> 1292 hgt 66 bmr<u>M</u> 1389 bmr<u>F</u> 1301
hgt 68 bmr<u>M</u> 1414 bmr<u>F</u> 1310 hgt 70 bmr<u>M</u> 1440 bmr<u>F</u> 1320
hgt 72 bmr<u>M</u> 1465 bmr<u>F</u> 1329 hgt 74 bmr<u>M</u> 1490 bmr<u>F</u> 1338
hgt 76 bmr<u>M</u> 1516 bmr<u>F</u> 1347 hgt 78 bmr<u>M</u> 1541 bmr<u>F</u> 1356

weight 170

hgt 60 bmr<u>M</u> 1375 bmr<u>F</u> 1317 hgt 62 bmr<u>M</u> 1400 bmr<u>F</u> 1327
hgt 64 bmr<u>M</u> 1426 bmr<u>F</u> 1336 hgt 66 bmr<u>M</u> 1451 bmr<u>F</u> 1345
hgt 68 bmr<u>M</u> 1476 bmr<u>F</u> 1354 hgt 70 bmr<u>M</u> 1502 bmr<u>F</u> 1363
hgt 72 bmr<u>M</u> 1527 bmr<u>F</u> 1372 hgt 74 bmr<u>M</u> 1553 bmr<u>F</u> 1381
hgt 76 bmr<u>M</u> 1578 bmr<u>F</u> 1391 hgt 78 bmr<u>M</u> 1603 bmr<u>F</u> 1400

weight 180

hgt 60 bmr<u>M</u> 1437 bmr<u>F</u> 1361   hgt 62 bmr<u>M</u> 1462 bmr<u>F</u> 1370
hgt 64 bmr<u>M</u> 1488 bmr<u>F</u> 1379   hgt 66 bmr<u>M</u> 1513 bmr<u>F</u> 1388
hgt 68 bmr<u>M</u> 1539 bmr<u>F</u> 1398   hgt 70 bmr<u>M</u> 1564 bmr<u>F</u> 1407
hgt 72 bmr<u>M</u> 1589 bmr<u>F</u> 1416   hgt 74 bmr<u>M</u> 1615 bmr<u>F</u> 1425
hgt 76 bmr<u>M</u> 1640 bmr<u>F</u> 1434   hgt 78 bmr<u>M</u> 1666 bmr<u>F</u> 1443

weight 190

hgt 60 bmr<u>M</u> 1499 bmr<u>F</u> 1405   hgt 62 bmr<u>M</u> 1525 bmr<u>F</u> 1414
hgt 64 bmr<u>M</u> 1550 bmr<u>F</u> 1423   hgt 66 bmr<u>M</u> 1575 bmr<u>F</u> 1432
hgt 68 bmr<u>M</u> 1601 bmr<u>F</u> 1441   hgt 70 bmr<u>M</u> 1626 bmr<u>F</u> 1450
hgt 72 bmr<u>M</u> 1652 bmr<u>F</u> 1459   hgt 74 bmr<u>M</u> 1677 bmr<u>F</u> 1469
hgt 76 bmr<u>M</u> 1702 bmr<u>F</u> 1478   hgt 78 bmr<u>M</u> 1728 bmr<u>F</u> 1487

weight 200

hgt 60 bmr<u>M</u> 1561 bmr<u>F</u> 1448   hgt 62 bmr<u>M</u> 1587 bmr<u>F</u> 1457
hgt 64 bmr<u>M</u> 1612 bmr<u>F</u> 1466   hgt 66 bmr<u>M</u> 1638 bmr<u>F</u> 1476
hgt 68 bmr<u>M</u> 1663 bmr<u>F</u> 1485   hgt 70 bmr<u>M</u> 1688 bmr<u>F</u> 1494
hgt 72 bmr<u>M</u> 1714 bmr<u>F</u> 1503   hgt 74 bmr<u>M</u> 1739 bmr<u>F</u> 1512
hgt 76 bmr<u>M</u> 1765 bmr<u>F</u> 1521   hgt 78 bmr<u>M</u> 1790 bmr<u>F</u> 1530

weight 210

hgt 60 bmr<u>M</u> 1624 bmr<u>F</u> 1492   hgt 62 bmr<u>M</u> 1649 bmr<u>F</u> 1501
hgt 64 bmr<u>M</u> 1674 bmr<u>F</u> 1510   hgt 66 bmr<u>M</u> 1700 bmr<u>F</u> 1519
hgt 68 bmr<u>M</u> 1725 bmr<u>F</u> 1528   hgt 70 bmr<u>M</u> 1751 bmr<u>F</u> 1538
hgt 72 bmr<u>M</u> 1776 bmr<u>F</u> 1547   hgt 74 bmr<u>M</u> 1801 bmr<u>F</u> 1556
hgt 76 bmr<u>M</u> 1827 bmr<u>F</u> 1565   hgt 78 bmr<u>M</u> 1852 bmr<u>F</u> 1574

weight 220

hgt 60 bmr<u>M</u> 1686 bmr<u>F</u> 1535   hgt 62 bmr<u>M</u> 1711 bmr<u>F</u> 1545
hgt 64 bmr<u>M</u> 1737 bmr<u>F</u> 1554   hgt 66 bmr<u>M</u> 1762 bmr<u>F</u> 1563
hgt 68 bmr<u>M</u> 1787 bmr<u>F</u> 1572   hgt 70 bmr<u>M</u> 1813 bmr<u>F</u> 1581
hgt 72 bmr<u>M</u> 1838 bmr<u>F</u> 1590   hgt 74 bmr<u>M</u> 1864 bmr<u>F</u> 1599
hgt 76 bmr<u>M</u> 1889 bmr<u>F</u> 1609   hgt 78 bmr<u>M</u> 1914 bmr<u>F</u> 1618

weight 230

hgt 60 bmr<u>M</u> 1748 bmr<u>F</u> 1579   hgt 62 bmr<u>M</u> 1773 bmr<u>F</u> 1588
hgt 64 bmr<u>M</u> 1799 bmr<u>F</u> 1597   hgt 66 bmr<u>M</u> 1824 bmr<u>F</u> 1606
hgt 68 bmr<u>M</u> 1850 bmr<u>F</u> 1616   hgt 70 bmr<u>M</u> 1875 bmr<u>F</u> 1625
hgt 72 bmr<u>M</u> 1900 bmr<u>F</u> 1634   hgt 74 bmr<u>M</u> 1926 bmr<u>F</u> 1643
hgt 76 bmr<u>M</u> 1951 bmr<u>F</u> 1652   hgt 78 bmr<u>M</u> 1977 bmr<u>F</u> 1661

<u>weight</u> 240

hgt 60 bmr<u>M</u> 1810 bmr<u>F</u> 1623   hgt 62 bmr<u>M</u> 1836 bmr<u>F</u> 1632
hgt 64 bmr<u>M</u> 1861 bmr<u>F</u> 1641   hgt 66 bmr<u>M</u> 1886 bmr<u>F</u> 1650
hgt 68 bmr<u>M</u> 1912 bmr<u>F</u> 1659   hgt 70 bmr<u>M</u> 1937 bmr<u>F</u> 1668
hgt 72 bmr<u>M</u> 1963 bmr<u>F</u> 1677   hgt 74 bmr<u>M</u> 1988 bmr<u>F</u> 1687
hgt 76 bmr<u>M</u> 2013 bmr<u>F</u> 1696   hgt 78 bmr<u>M</u> 2039 bmr<u>F</u> 1705

<u>weight</u> 250

hgt 60 bmr<u>M</u> 1872 bmr<u>F</u> 1666   hgt 62 bmr<u>M</u> 1898 bmr<u>F</u> 1675
hgt 64 bmr<u>M</u> 1923 bmr<u>F</u> 1684   hgt 66 bmr<u>M</u> 1949 bmr<u>F</u> 1694
hgt 68 bmr<u>M</u> 1974 bmr<u>F</u> 1703   hgt 70 bmr<u>M</u> 1999 bmr<u>F</u> 1712
hgt 72 bmr<u>M</u> 2025 bmr<u>F</u> 1721   hgt 74 bmr<u>M</u> 2050 bmr<u>F</u> 1730
hgt 76 bmr<u>M</u> 2076 bmr<u>F</u> 1739   hgt 78 bmr<u>M</u> 2101 bmr<u>F</u> 1748

<u>weight</u> 260

hgt 60 bmr<u>M</u> 1935 bmr<u>F</u> 1710   hgt 62 bmr<u>M</u> 1960 bmr<u>F</u> 1719
hgt 64 bmr<u>M</u> 1985 bmr<u>F</u> 1728   hgt 66 bmr<u>M</u> 2011 bmr<u>F</u> 1737
hgt 68 bmr<u>M</u> 2036 bmr<u>F</u> 1746   hgt 70 bmr<u>M</u> 2062 bmr<u>F</u> 1756
hgt 72 bmr<u>M</u> 2087 bmr<u>F</u> 1765   hgt 74 bmr<u>M</u> 2112 bmr<u>F</u> 1774
hgt 76 bmr<u>M</u> 2138 bmr<u>F</u> 1783   hgt 78 bmr<u>M</u> 2163 bmr<u>F</u> 1792

<u>weight</u> 270

hgt 60 bmr<u>M</u> 1997 bmr<u>F</u> 1753   hgt 62 bmr<u>M</u> 2022 bmr<u>F</u> 1763
hgt 64 bmr<u>M</u> 2048 bmr<u>F</u> 1772   hgt 66 bmr<u>M</u> 2073 bmr<u>F</u> 1781
hgt 68 bmr<u>M</u> 2098 bmr<u>F</u> 1790   hgt 70 bmr<u>M</u> 2124 bmr<u>F</u> 1799
hgt 72 bmr<u>M</u> 2149 bmr<u>F</u> 1808   hgt 74 bmr<u>M</u> 2175 bmr<u>F</u> 1817
hgt 76 bmr<u>M</u> 2200 bmr<u>F</u> 1827   hgt 78 bmr<u>M</u> 2225 bmr<u>F</u> 1836

<u>weight</u> 280

hgt 60 bmr<u>M</u> 2059 bmr<u>F</u> 1797   hgt 62 bmr<u>M</u> 2084 bmr<u>F</u> 1806
hgt 64 bmr<u>M</u> 2110 bmr<u>F</u> 1815   hgt 66 bmr<u>M</u> 2135 bmr<u>F</u> 1824
hgt 68 bmr<u>M</u> 2161 bmr<u>F</u> 1834   hgt 70 bmr<u>M</u> 2186 bmr<u>F</u> 1843
hgt 72 bmr<u>M</u> 2211 bmr<u>F</u> 1852   hgt 74 bmr<u>M</u> 2237 bmr<u>F</u> 1861
hgt 76 bmr<u>M</u> 2262 bmr<u>F</u> 1870   hgt 78 bmr<u>M</u> 2288 bmr<u>F</u> 1879

<u>weight</u> 290

hgt 60 bmr<u>M</u> 2121 bmr<u>F</u> 1841   hgt 62 bmr<u>M</u> 2147 bmr<u>F</u> 1850
hgt 64 bmr<u>M</u> 2172 bmr<u>F</u> 1859   hgt 66 bmr<u>M</u> 2197 bmr<u>F</u> 1868
hgt 68 bmr<u>M</u> 2223 bmr<u>F</u> 1877   hgt 70 bmr<u>M</u> 2248 bmr<u>F</u> 1886
hgt 72 bmr<u>M</u> 2274 bmr<u>F</u> 1895   hgt 74 bmr<u>M</u> 2299 bmr<u>F</u> 1905
hgt 76 bmr<u>M</u> 2324 bmr<u>F</u> 1914   hgt 78 bmr<u>M</u> 2350 bmr<u>F</u> 1923

<u>weight</u> 300

hgt 60 bmr<u>M</u> 2183 bmr<u>F</u> 1884 hgt 62 bmr<u>M</u> 2209 bmr<u>F</u> 1893
hgt 64 bmr<u>M</u> 2234 bmr<u>F</u> 1902 hgt 66 bmr<u>M</u> 2260 bmr<u>F</u> 1912
hgt 68 bmr<u>M</u> 2285 bmr<u>F</u> 1921 hgt 70 bmr<u>M</u> 2310 bmr<u>F</u> 1930
hgt 72 bmr<u>M</u> 2336 bmr<u>F</u> 1939 hgt 74 bmr<u>M</u> 2361 bmr<u>F</u> 1948
hgt 76 bmr<u>M</u> 2387 bmr<u>F</u> 1957 hgt 78 bmr<u>M</u> 2412 bmr<u>F</u> 1966

References

American Heart Association
http://www.justmove.org/myfitness/actarticles/acframes.cfm?Target=hartrates.html

Bullough, R, Gillette C, Harris M, and Melby C. Interaction of acute changes in exercise energy expenditure and energy intake on resting metabolic rate. *Am J Clin Nutr* 61: 473-481, 1995

Fukagawa, NK, Bandini LG, and Young JB. Effect of age on body composition and resting metabolic rate. *Am J Physiol Endocrinol Metab* 259: E233-E238, 1990.

Horber, FF, Kohler SA, Lippuner K, and Jaeger P. Effect of regular physical training on age-associated alterations in body composition in men. *Eur J Clin Invest* 26: 279-285, 1996

Layton, Julia. "How Calories Work"
http://www.howstuffworks.com/calorie3.htm

Leonard S. Piers, Mario J. Soares, Leanne M. McCormack and Kaerin O'dea Is there evidence for an age-related reduction in metabolic rate? *J Appl Physiol* 85: 2196-2204, 1998

http://www.nutrition.gov

Pollock, ML, Mengelkock LJ, Graves JE, Lowenthal DT, Limacher MC, Foster C, and Wilmore JH. Twenty-year follow-up of aerobic power and body composition of older track athletes. *J Appl Physiol* 82: 1508-1516, 1997

J Polivy. Psychological consequences of food restriction. Journal of the American Dietetic Association 96: 6(JUN 1996): 589-592.

YOYO Diets cause heart disease by lowering HDL. *Journal of the American College of Cardiology November, 2000*; 36: 1565-1571

Ballor DL, Harvey-Berino JR, Ades PA, Cryan J, Calles-Escandon J. Contrasting effects of resistance and aerobic training on body composition and metabolism after diet-induced weight loss. Metabolism. 1996;45:179-183.

http://www.nal.usda.gov/fnic/foodcomp/srch/search.htm

http://www.nutrition.gov/index.php?mode=subject&subject=ng_composition&d_subject=Food%20Com position

http://www.nal.usda.gov/fnic/foodcomp/srch/search.htm

ED. Shade, CM. Ulrich, MH. Wener, et al. Frequent intentional weight loss is associated with lower natural killer cell cytotoxicity in postmenopausal women: possible long-term immune effects. J Am Diet Assoc. 2004, vol. 104, pp. 903--912

Index:

aerobic, 93, 94, 95, 97, 98, 99, 123, 127, 129, 130, 137, 161
aerobic exercise, 94, 95, 97, 98, 99, 123, 127
anaerobic, 94, 95, 98, 99, 127, 130, 137
anaerobic exercise, 94, 95, 99, 127, 130, 137
BMR, 3, 15, 16, 22, 23, 24, 26, 27, 28, 29, 30, 33, 37, 94, 126, 129, 136, 138, 157, 159, 160, 161
body fat, 6, 10, 16, 27, 29, 30, 36, 56, 94, 95, 97, 98, 127, 129, 131, 136, 144, 157, 158
body weight, 9, 10, 14, 26, 29, 31, 90, 129, 136, 143
caloric, 4, 7, 10, 11, 14, 24, 26, 27, 29, 30, 32, 33, 35, 38, 50, 51, 52, 53, 54, 58, 60, 64, 66, 70, 85, 90, 94, 128, 130, 131, 133, 134, 136, 137, 140, 142, 149, 156, 160
calorie, 28, 126, 160
calorie counter, 27, 35, 51, 56, 145, 155
calories, 4, 6, 7, 9, 10, 11, 14, 15, 16, 19, 22, 23, 25, 26, 27, 29, 30, 31, 32, 33, 35, 36, 37, 41, 42, 46, 47, 48, 49, 50, 51, 52, 53, 54, 55, 56, 57, 58, 59, 60, 61, 62, 63, 64, 65, 66, 67, 68, 69, 70, 71, 72, 73, 74, 75, 76, 77, 78, 79, 80, 81, 82, 83, 84, 85, 86, 87, 88, 89, 90,
93, 94, 95, 97, 99, 100, 123, 125, 126, 127, 128, 129, 130, 131, 132, 133, 134, 136, 137, 138, 139, 140, 141, 144, 145, 146, 148, 149, 155, 156, 157, 160
daily dieting, 4, 5, 15, 16, 24, 30, 31
DCN, 26, 27, 29, 30, 31, 32, 33, 34, 35, 36, 37, 53, 99, 126, 127, 128, 129, 130, 133, 134, 135, 136, 137, 138, 139, 141, 144, 145, 147, 155, 157
exercise, 6, 9, 10, 11, 19, 21, 22, 26, 28, 30, 33, 36, 39, 51, 93, 94, 95, 97, 98, 99, 100, 103, 105, 123, 124, 125, 126, 127, 128, 129, 130, 134, 137, 139, 142, 160, 161
full-day, 30, 34, 37, 128, 129, 130, 131, 133, 134, 135, 137, 138, 140, 143
full-days, 30, 37, 129, 130, 131, 134, 137, 138, 140, 143
genetic background, 27
glycemic index, 55
Harris Benedict Formula, 27
Internet, 27, 29, 51, 133
legal cheating, 142, 145
light-day, 30, 31, 32, 34, 35, 36, 37, 127, 128, 130, 131, 133, 134, 135, 137, 138, 139, 143, 144

light-days, 30, 31, 32, 34, 35,
36, 37, 127, 128, 130, 131,
133, 137, 139, 143, 144
maintenance, 5, 30, 40, 97,
127, 135, 142, 145, 146,
147, 157
metabolism, 6, 15, 130, 133,
141, 161
multiplier, 28, 98, 126, 130,
138, 160
muscle, 6, 7, 10, 15, 16, 19,
27, 29, 30, 31, 33, 37, 93,
94, 95, 96, 97, 99, 123, 127,
129, 131, 136, 144, 147, 157
plateau, 4, 13, 16, 29, 30, 31,
36, 37, 99, 134, 135, 139,
140
PRE, 95, 96, 98, 99
PREs, 96, 99
stretching, 25, 124
vacation week, 138, 144
WCN, 26, 27, 30, 31, 37